AF262872

HEALTHY LIVING

High-Protein Cookbook

85 Recipes and Meal Plans to Build Muscle, Balance Metabolism, and Thrive at Any Age

TOBY AMIDOR MS RD

For my three children—Schoen, Ellena, and Micah—
you are the constant catalysts for my personal growth.
I love you.

This book is also dedicated to everyone who seeks to improve their health through the power of protein. You deserve to feel your best.

Healthy Living High-Protein Cookbook

Published by Cider Mill Press, an imprint of HarperCollins Focus LLC, 501 Nelson Place, Nashville, TN 37214 USA.

13-Digit ISBN: 978-1-40035-524-2
10-Digit ISBN: 1-40035-524-9

Books published by Cider Mill Press Book Publishers are available at special discounts for bulk purchases in the United States by corporations, institutions, and other organizations. For more information, please contact the publisher.

cidermillpress.com

HarperCollins Publishers, Macken House, 39/40 Mayor Street Upper, Dublin1, D01C9W8, Ireland (https://www.harpercollins.com)

Typography: New Spirit by Newlyn and Polymath by OH no Type Co.

Image Credits: Cover photo and photos on pages 116, 172, 188, and 200 used under official license from StockFood.com; photo on pages viii–1 from Pexels.com; photos on pages 136, 226–227, 240–241, 250 used under official license from Adobe Stock. All other photos used are under official license from Shutterstock.com. Background textures from texturelabs.org.

Printed in Malaysia

26 27 28 29 30 SEA 5 4 3 2 1

First Edition

Contents

Introduction

I have been working as a registered dietitian for twenty-five years, and I love carbs. Yes, carbs. I know you opened this book wanting to read about protein, but I just can't deny my love for carbs. So, what's the problem with being a carb-lover? If I want my body to work as efficiently as possible, I can't eat all the carbs I want and love. I need to choose my carbs carefully and balance them with healthy fat and protein. This has become especially important since I reached the age of fifty and have begun to feel the natural changes that occur with age.

Throughout my life I have experienced the many changes in the human body. At age forty, I gained some weight but was able to lose it by balancing my diet, incorporating enough protein, exercising regularly, and maintaining an overall healthy lifestyle. But now at fifty, in the middle of perimenopause, I gained even more weight due to my life phase and decline of estrogen, and am in need of a bit more protein to help maintain my muscle mass. My protein needs are even greater because I also play competitive USTA tennis on about nine teams throughout the year and even captain a few of them. This means that I am on the tennis courts at least four days—if not more—every week. I also practice reformer Pilates and hike with my dogs regularly. Protein certainly plays an important role in my diet, helping to keep my body in tip-top shape.

Although I don't practice privately anymore, I do help friends who ask me for guidance. A few years ago, a physician I dated wanted to lose about twenty pounds, and he was committed to making healthy changes in his life. At the beginning of his weight loss journey, he texted and called me regularly asking me nutrition questions and wanting help selecting healthier choices at each meal. Protein played a huge role in my guidance. I educated him on better protein choices, portion sizes, and also the proper way to eat protein throughout the day for maximum efficiency and balanced meals. Ultimately, it took him about six months to lose the weight, which aligns with the National Institutes of Health's recommendation for healthy weight loss of one to two pounds per week. He's also kept the weight off for nearly two years and now makes his own healthy choices and understands what his body needs.

But nutrition isn't always as straightforward as "eat more protein," and that really isn't what this cookbook is about. As I mentioned above, *when* you eat protein is the big secret. Regardless of how much the media may recommend it or you may hear your friends and family say that they are trying to eat loads of protein, it's important to understand that more isn't necessarily better.

Over the past twenty years as a registered dietitian, I have seen nutrition fads come and go, and today, misinformation is at its peak due to the rapid speed at which information spreads on social media. Looking back at my freshman year in college in the 1990s, low fat was all the rage—everyone in my dorm stocked up on "fat-free" Snackwell's cookies. That fad came in strong and passed within a few years. Over time, however, we began to recognize that fat plays an important role in the diet, and recommendations evolved to emphasize eating "healthy fats." With meat and poultry, the focus shifted toward choosing lean protein with less saturated fat.

When it comes to protein, a lot of misinformation is swirling around. High-protein diets, which began with the Atkins Diet, have been popular over the past few decades. The founder of the diet, Dr. Atkins, was the original ketogenic diet advocate; he recommended cutting out most carbs and focusing on protein and fat as a fuel for energy. The funny thing is that Dr. Atkins never meant for someone to stay on the ketogenic diet forever. In the last section of his diet plan, he recommends adding carbs back into the diet. Interestingly, when the keto diet was at its peak popularity, people were convinced they needed to stay in a ketogenic state (a state where your body's energy is fueled by fat and not carbs) in order to lose weight and stay healthy. However, most people realized that the diet wasn't sustainable long term and that sipping on olive oil and eating meat, eggs, fish, or chicken all day really wasn't tasty. If you take away one piece of advice from this book, make it this: Every meal you eat—especially healthy meals balanced with protein—should always be tasty!

Today, protein is a hot topic. The 2025 International Food Information Council's Food and Health Survey found that people are as keen on protein as ever. The survey also found that, for the fifth straight year, protein is the nutrient Americans say they are most focused on consuming. And for the third straight year, a high-protein diet is the most common eating pattern Americans are following. Interestingly, the survey also found that 2025 marks the first time a "good source of protein"—a label you can find on food packaging—is the most common criterion Americans use to define a healthy food[1].

So, how will protein fit into your healthy eating plan? Whether you're looking to build muscle mass, lose weight, maintain weight, or just become healthier overall, protein plays an important part of your diet. In this book, you'll find science-based information from a credible registered dietitian (that's me!) with a master's degree in clinical nutrition and dietetics from New York University. I have spent my career doing a "salad" of things, including educating chefs about nutrition, mentoring new registered dietitians trained at various universities, counseling clients, and educating consumers through my media writing, helping them cut through misinformation and providing information backed by credible scientific research.

Within the first three chapters of this book, I break down what protein is and its many roles in the body. In addition, because everyone has individual needs, I discuss different protein requirements depending on who you are, what your goals are, and how you prefer to consume your daily protein. (Hint: it's all about *when* you eat your protein and *how much*.) I also dispel numerous myths about protein—please do sit down before reading that section!

In chapter 2, I discuss the various sources of protein. Although I am omnivorous (I eat both plant and animal foods), I include information about protein that those following a vegetarian eating plan should know. And, with grocery prices at an all-time high, I also share budget-friendly protein tips, easy higher-protein swaps, and one of my favorite topics—meal prepping.

I also want to set you up for success. That's where chapter 3 comes in: You'll find information on cooking and planning for protein success. This includes techniques for preparing various animal and plant proteins, as well as guidance on proper internal cooking temperatures. The recipes throughout this cookbook indicate doneness using internal cooking temperatures, as this is the most reliable way to ensure your food is fully cooked. You'll find a section on purchasing the best thermometers too.

And don't worry! I didn't forget about snacks. These mini-meals are an important part of meeting your daily protein goals. You'll find guidance on the ideal amount of protein to include in a snack, as well as which foods can help fill some of the nutrient gaps common among Americans.

At the end of chapter 3, you'll find four one-week meal plans. The first is designed for a woman in perimenopause who is an omnivore and eats animal and plant proteins and exercises 45 minutes, 3 to 4 days a week. The second is for a woman in postmenopause who is a vegetarian and exercises 45 minutes, 3 to 4 days a week. The third is designed for an adult man who is an omnivore and exercises 1 hour, 4 to 5 days a week. The last is designed for an adult woman who is an omnivore and exercises most days of the week for 1 hour. All the meal plans are balanced with carbs and fat. I've provided both because everyone has individual goals and eating preferences. As I always say: you do you!

When you get to the recipe chapters, you'll find that each recipe provides a lot of useful information. And, importantly, every recipe uses easily accessible ingredients that don't break the bank. I know what it is like to cook for a family or even for one or two people—it takes a lot of time and planning—so I've tried to provide simple yet tasty recipes that are easy to cook.

Every recipe identifies whether it is vegan, vegetarian, gluten-free, and/or dairy-free. I also indicate if a recipe is freezer-friendly, good for meal prepping, can be whipped up in thirty minutes or less, and if it is a one-pot or one-pan meal (something I always look for in recipes!).

Each recipe lists the number of servings and the serving size. It's easy to serve yourself as much as you can fit on a plate or what feels like the right portion, but that may not match the calories and protein listed in the recipe. After making the dish, measuring the correct portion size is essential to ensure you're getting the amount of protein you want. You'll also find nutrition information for each recipe, including calories, total fat, saturated fat, protein, total carbohydrates, fiber, total and added sugars, and sodium. Everyone values different information, so I wanted it all at your fingertips. Lastly, each recipe includes one "Toby's Tip," where I offer substitutions, complementary recipes, and other culinary or nutrition information you may find useful.

I recommend trying a handful of recipes that look appealing, and if they're a hit, add them to your weeknight rotation. Most people rotate about ten recipes in their regular repertoire, so I hope you use this opportunity to swap some of your older, lower-protein dishes out for some new ones or use the tips in this cookbook to boost the protein in some of your tried-and-true favorites.

In this cookbook, I've aimed to make your life as easy as possible by providing useful information and recipes that are higher in protein, tasty, budget-friendly, and simple to prepare. I can't wait for you to dig into this protein-rich content and get started on your journey toward better protein intake within your balanced diet and overall health.

I wish you lifelong healthy, happy, and protein-filled eating.

—Toby

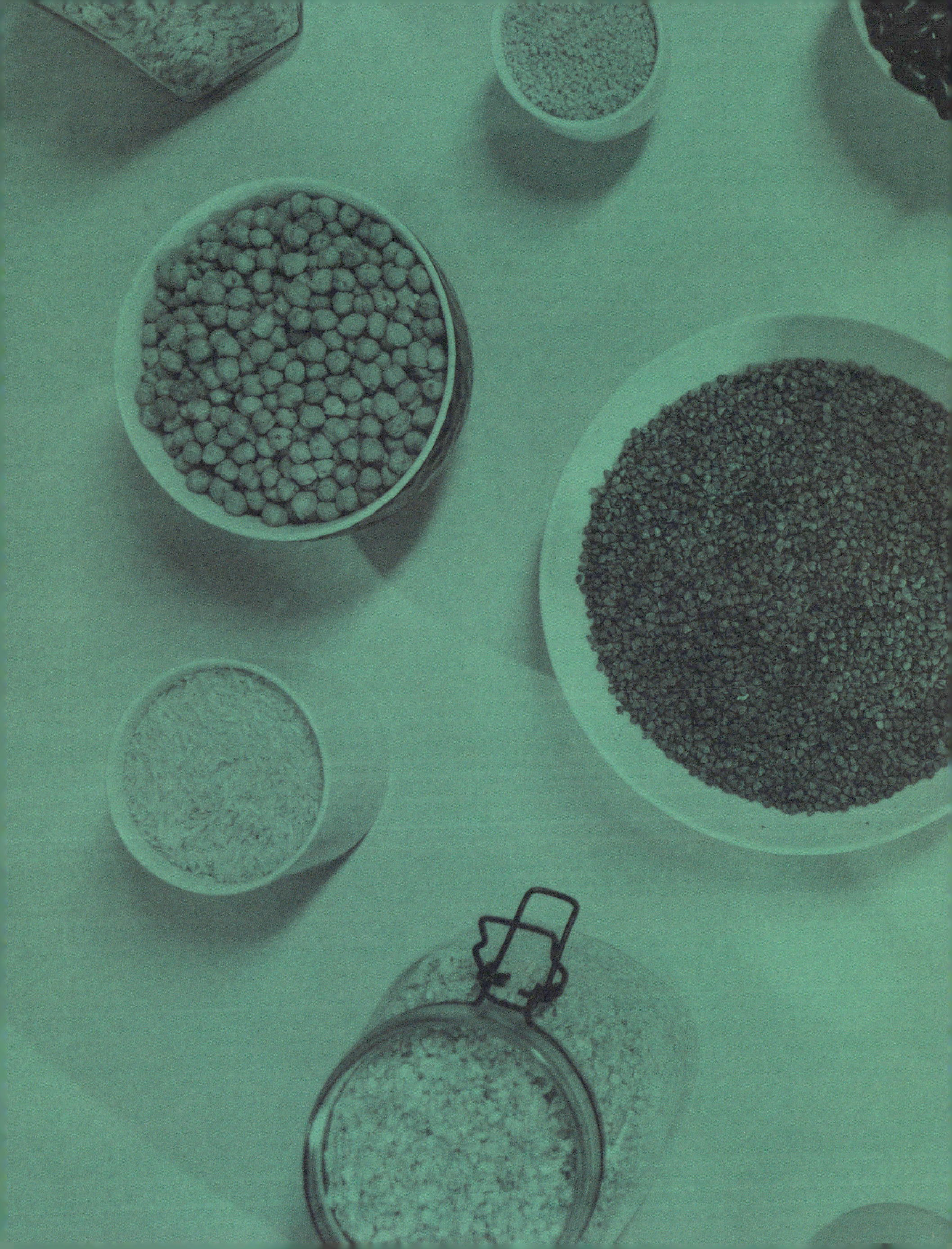

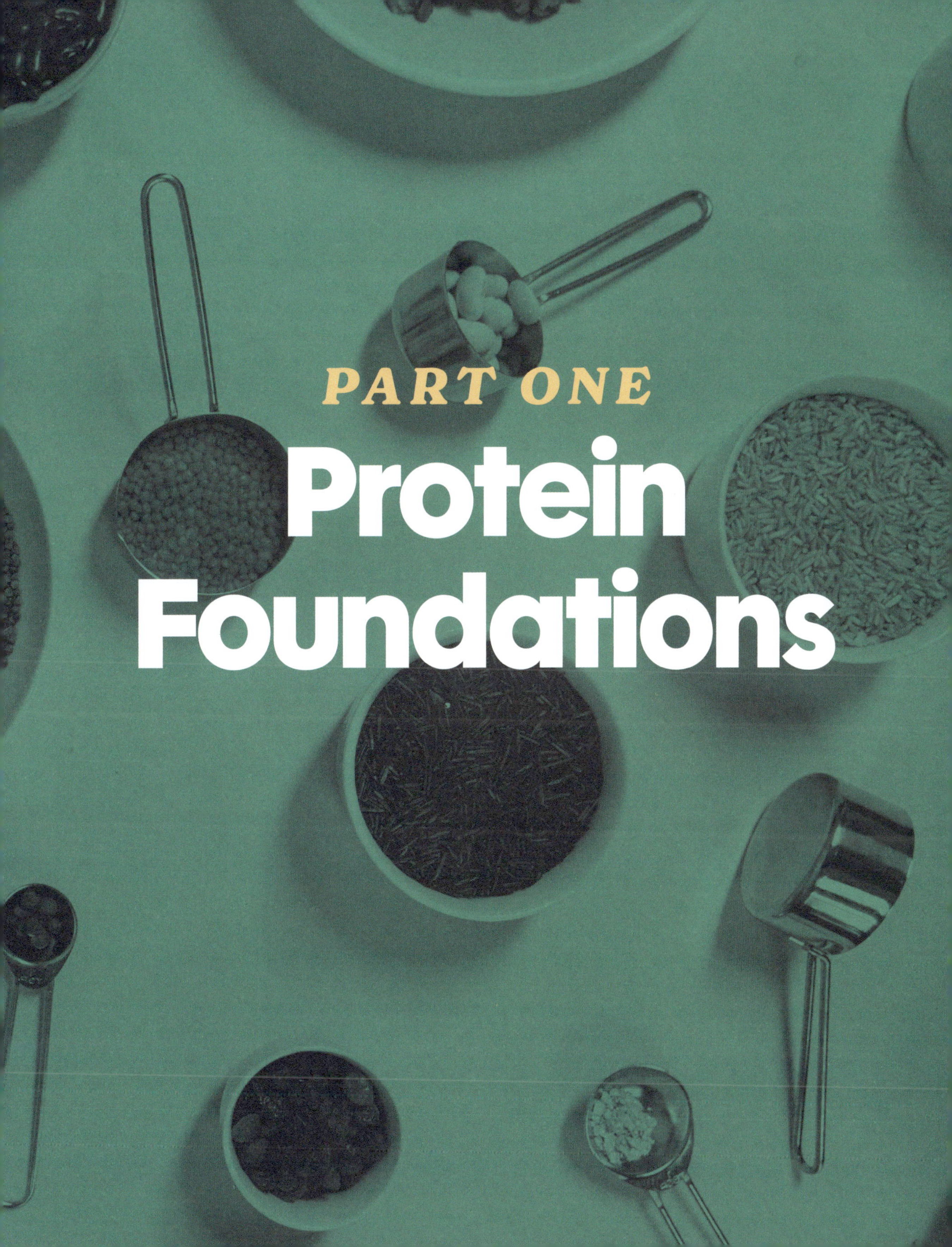

PART ONE

Protein Foundations

CHAPTER 1

Strength and Satiety: *Why Protein Matters*

The Science of Protein

Protein is one of three essential macronutrients, along with carbohydrates and fat. Understanding protein on a structural level (don't worry, I won't get too technical) and the various roles it plays in your body is important for gaining a solid understanding of how foods support your body in staying healthy.

So, let's start with the chemistry. Protein is similar to carbohydrates and fat, as they are all made from carbon, hydrogen, and oxygen. However, unlike the other macros, protein contains nitrogen and provides much of the body's nitrogen.

The building blocks of protein are amino acids. Proteins are formed when long chains of amino acids are linked together. The specific order of the amino acids within these chains determines the protein's structure and function. There are twenty amino acids in total, nine of which are essential, meaning the body cannot produce them or cannot produce them in sufficient amounts. These essential amino acids must be obtained through food. The remaining eleven amino acids are considered non-essential because the body can synthesize them. However, under certain circumstances (such as illness), the body may not produce enough of these nonessential amino acids. In these cases, they are referred to as conditionally essential amino acids.

I won't list all of the amino acids because you don't select protein based on individual amino acids. Rather, it's best to eat a variety of proteins to ensure you take in a full range of amino acids that your body needs.

When amino acids connect to each other, they form a peptide bond. Protein fragments with ten or more amino acids are called polypeptides. Your body contains more than fifty thousand different proteins, each with a unique number and sequence of amino acid. This number and sequences of amino acids in a protein chain is called its primary structure. However, proteins cannot function in the body as long, straight chains. Instead, the protein chain bends in different ways, forming what is called the protein's secondary structure. Then the chain folds and twists further, creating its tertiary structure. Imagine a coiled cord—like the old-school phone cords from phones that plugged into the wall. The way a protein folds and twists allows it to function properly. This also helps explain why protein takes longer to digest. The body must unravel and break down these complex structures into their basic amino acids, a process that takes extra time. As a result, eating protein leaves you feeling fuller because of all the work your body does to break it down.

Protein has many functions in the body, as do carbohydrates and fat. That is why a balanced diet is essential, so you can get everything your body needs to support all its functions. Here are nine important roles that protein plays in your body:

1. PROTEIN IS PART OF THE BODY'S STRUCTURE.

Protein is critical to maintaining the elasticity and shape of cells and tissues in the body. You can find protein in muscles, but also in many other places in the body, such as your bones, hair, skin, fingernails, blood vessels, blood, and the digestive tract.

2. PROTEIN IS USED FOR BUILDING AND MAINTAINING THE BODY'S TISSUES.

Found in every cell, protein has been called the building block of life. Most of the body's cells are constantly broken down and rebuilt, including the protein within them. For example, the cells lining your gastrointestinal system are replaced every few days, and skin cells live for only about thirty days. In addition, during pregnancy or periods of growth, the body is continuously building new tissue. Protein is also needed to help repair tissue that is lost or damaged, such as during infection, burns, surgery, or age-related loss of muscle mass.

3. PROTEIN HELPS CELLS COMMUNICATE.

Protein is a component of some hormones, which are chemical messengers that help the body communicate. Hormones also regulate certain bodily activities, helping maintain homeostasis—a constant internal environment—such as body temperature.

4. PROTEIN IS A COMPONENT OF MANY ENZYMES.

Enzymes help speed up numerous reactions in the body. For example, they aid in breaking down food and in building substances such as bone and muscle.

5. PROTEIN IS A PART OF ALL ANTIBODIES.

If you're looking to support your immune system, adequate protein is essential. Antibodies are blood proteins whose job is to attach to foreign invaders—such as bacteria, viruses, and toxins—and help destroy them.

6. PROTEIN ACTS AS A TRANSPORTER THROUGHOUT THE BODY.

Your blood carries oxygen from your lungs to the rest of your body, and protein is needed to produce the cells that do this. Other substances—such as minerals, certain vitamins, fats, and oxygen—are also carried through the blood by various protein cells.

7. PROTEIN HELPS YOUR BLOOD CLOT.

When you cut yourself, protein fibers help form a clot so you stop bleeding.

8. PROTEIN HELPS MAINTAIN FLUID BALANCE AND ACID-BASE BALANCE.

Your body maintains fluid balance by attracting and retaining water in the bloodstream, preventing excess fluid from moving into tissues and causing swelling (known as edema). In addition, your body is constantly maintaining its proper pH, balancing foods and other processes in your body that produce acids and bases.

9. PROTEIN PROVIDES ENERGY.

Protein serves as an energy source when needed. Protein provides four calories per gram.

Who Needs a Higher-Protein Diet—and Why

Depending on age, activity level, and health, some people need more protein than others.

AGE

Perimenopausal women have increased protein needs due to declining muscle mass and a slower metabolism, which can lead to weight gain—protein can help regulate metabolism and promote satiety, as well as support bone health. In addition, post-menopausal and older adults require more protein to help prevent sarcopenia, the age-related loss of muscle mass and strength. Consuming more protein daily can help preserve muscle mass, mobility, function, and overall movement.

ACTIVITY LEVEL

People who are more active need more protein, especially athletes. If you strength train regularly (e.g., lift weights), your protein needs go up in order to build and repair muscle tissues. If you're training for endurance sports (e.g., running a marathon), you also have higher calorie and protein needs in order to fuel these long activities and help prevent your muscles from breaking down for energy. Those who regularly participate in high-intensity activities can also benefit from more protein in their diet. For example, playing competitive tennis for at least two hours a day, four days a week, over nearly twenty years—as I have—or engaging in high-intensity interval training (HIIT) like Orange Theory Fitness, which I also did three to four days a week, can raise your protein needs. Occasional high-intensity exercise doesn't significantly change your protein requirements; it's the consistent, long-term activity that matters.

HEALTH

Someone who is sick or has certain health conditions may need more protein. Individuals who are critically ill, have severe burns, have undergone major surgery, or are fighting infections typically require extra protein to repair tissue, preserve muscle, and support a stronger immune response during recovery. In addition, people with wasting diseases that cause unintentional weight loss—such as cancer, AIDS, and malnourishment—deplete the body's protein stores, and increased protein can help combat muscle wasting. Finally, those with chronic wounds or major injuries need higher protein intake to support the healing process.

It's important to note that some health conditions require less protein. For example, individuals with chronic kidney disease may not tolerate high amounts of protein, as it can put strain on the kidneys. That's why it's essential to consult your healthcare provider, especially when you're ill, about individual protein needs.

LIFE STAGE

Pregnant women need more protein to support fetal growth and development, while breastfeeding women need more protein to support milk production, tissue repair, and the infant's development. Infants, toddlers, children, and teenagers need more protein in their diet to help support growth and development.

PROTEIN & HORMONAL HEALTH AFTER FORTY

After the age of forty, both men and women start losing significant amounts of skeletal muscle. However, starting around forty (or even in the late thirties) during perimenopause and menopause, protein is critical to help regulate hormones. During this time, estrogen levels begin to decline, which affects not only reproductive health but also bone density, muscle mass, and metabolic rate. As a result, more muscle protein is broken down while less is synthesized. This is why protein intake is more important at this age than ever—and why protein needs increase.

Another hormone, progesterone, also declines during this time, which can contribute to perimenopause symptoms such as poor sleep, mood swings, and elevated levels of the stress hormone cortisol. As I write this, I check off each of these symptoms in my own experience, and many of my friends in this stage of life report the same challenges. Including protein in your meals and snacks, as outlined in this book, can help stabilize blood sugar, reduce cortisol spikes, and support more stable mood.

Lastly, as you age and your hormones shift during perimenopause, your body becomes less efficient at managing blood sugar—so you may have reduced insulin sensitivity. Incorporating protein in the right amount throughout your meals and snacks can help slow the absorption of carbohydrates, which can help regulate blood sugar levels.

Once you hit the age of sixty, there is an increase in muscle being broken down. At this age, protein needs are still higher and weight-bearing exercises are highly encouraged.

During these times, your protein needs don't skyrocket. We aren't back in the 1980s, when commercials showed a huge rib-eye steak being served with three stalks of broccoli. Instead, your protein needs increase by a small to moderate amount, depending on factors like age and activity level. The key is how much protein you eat at each meal and snack throughout the day and taking in a variety of protein, so you get all the amino acids your body needs. In the chapter, I'll explain this concept so you can master it with proper planning and some practice.

How Much Protein Do You Really Need?

Protein needs vary throughout life and differ from person to person. This cookbook can help guide you in meeting your protein goals properly as a healthy adult. It also provides guidelines for individuals with higher protein needs after the age of forty, when skeletal muscle decline accelerates in perimenopause and postmenopausal women, as well as in men. After age sixty, muscle loss tends to speed up further for both men and women, increasing protein needs even more.

FOR A HEALTHY ADULT, UP TO AGE FORTY

The recommended dietary allowance (RDA) of protein to prevent deficiency in an average adult with low physical activity is 0.8 grams per kilogram of body weight, or 0.36 grams per pound per day.

- For a 150-pound healthy woman 18 and over (not in perimenopause), multiply 150 pounds × 0.36 grams per pound of body weight = **54 grams of protein per day.**

- For a 190-pound healthy man, multiply 190 pounds × 0.36 grams per pound of body weight = **68.4 grams of protein per day**.

FOR ADULTS OVER FORTY, OR IN PERIMENOPAUSE

Individuals who are over forty or in perimenopause and are sedentary or not meeting weekly recommendations for physical activity have higher protein requirements. During perimenopause and beyond, daily protein intake should increase to 1.0 to 1.2 grams per kilogram of body weight, or 0.45 to 0.54 grams per pound, per day. Being sedentary typically means spending at least six hours a day in low-activity behaviors, such as watching screens, driving, or sitting at a desk.

- For a sedentary woman over forty (in perimenopause) who weighs 150 pounds, multiply 150 pounds × 0.45 grams per pound of body weight = **67.5 grams of protein at the lower end** and 150 pounds × 0.54 grams per pound of body weight = **81 grams of protein at the higher end per day**.

If you are an active adult man or woman who meets the recommendations of exercising 60 to 90 minutes most days of the week, your protein requirements increase to 1.2 to 1.6 grams of protein per kilogram body weight or 0.54 to 0.72 grams per pound of body weight each day.

- For an active woman over forty (in perimenopause) who weighs 150 pounds, multiply 150 pounds × 0.54 grams per pound of body weight = **81 grams of protein at the lower end** and 150 pounds × 0.72 grams per pound of body weight **= 108 grams of protein at the higher end.**

If you are an adult man or woman who lifts weights or is training for a running or cycling event 5 to 7 days per week, your needs can be 1.2 to 1.7 grams per kilogram body weight or 0.54 to 0.77 grams per pound of body weight each day.

- For an active man over forty who weighs 200 pounds, multiply 200 pounds × 0.54 grams per pound of body weight = **108 grams of protein at the lower end** and 200 pounds × 0.77 grams per pound of body weight **= 154 grams of protein at the higher end.**

EXCESSIVE PROTEIN INTAKE

Excessive protein intake is typically more than 2 grams of protein per kilogram of body weight (or 0.9 grams of protein per pound of body weight) each day.

- For an active 150-pound woman over forty, this means 150 pounds × 0.9 grams per pound of body weight = **135 grams protein.**
- For an active 200-pound man over forty, this means 200 × 0.9 grams per pound of body weight = **180 grams protein.**

Note: Protein needs increase during pregnancy, breastfeeding, and throughout childhood and teenage years. This book targets healthy non-pregnant or non-breastfeeding adults and children. Consult your healthcare provider to determine your individual needs and enjoy the recipes in this cookbook.

Timing, Absorption, and Variety

If you're tempted to get all your protein by chugging a huge protein drink that contains 50 or 60 grams of protein, it's not recommended. Consuming too much of one food, like protein, means you may be missing out on other important foods and nutrients—and that is not beneficial for your body. Getting enough protein depends on several factors, including timing, absorption, and variety.

It's recommended to spread your protein intake throughout the day, across meals and snacks. This helps promote balanced meals, supports overall nutrition, and keeps you feeling satisfied longer. Typically, people consume the least amount of protein at breakfast and the most at dinner. But with the strategies in this book, you will change that!

Research shows that getting enough protein at breakfast, lunch, and dinner can help with weight management by helping you feel satisfied and decreasing cravings throughout the day. Current recommendations are to spread protein intake throughout the day (versus consuming large amounts all at once). It is recommended to consume between 15 to 30 grams of protein at every meal, and no more than 40 grams of protein at every meal. Consuming over 40 grams of protein can lead to an imbalance of other foods and nutrients.

For snacks, a good target is 10 to 15 grams of protein. Snacks act as mini meals that help fill nutrient gaps, including protein, and should include a combination of foods to maximize the nutrients you take in. Chapter 11 contains ten snack recipes that have higher amounts of protein per serving to help you reach your daily protein goals.

Also, the variety of protein matters. According to the 2020–2025 Dietary Guidelines for Americans, most individuals meet or come close to the daily recommended amount of protein per day (at 0.8 grams per kilograms body weight). However, protein can be obtained from a variety of foods across several subgroups. These subgroups include: 1) meat, poultry, and eggs; 2) seafood; 3) nuts, seeds, and soy products. Taking in a variety of protein sources means you also take in a wider variety of amino acids and nutrients that your body needs. Many Americans do not meet the recommended amount of protein from specific protein subgroups. According to the 2020–2025 Dietary Guidelines for Americans, about 75 percent of Americans meet or exceed the recommended amounts for meat, poultry and eggs. However, almost 90 percent don't meet the recommended amounts for seafood, and more than 50 percent don't meet the recommended amounts for nuts, seeds, and soy[2]. Chapter 2 covers what protein sources are included in each of these subgroups and why they are important.

Common Protein Myths

With protein being such a trendy topic and with the lightning speed of misinformation spreading on social media, there are many widespread misconceptions about protein. Here are the top eight myths about protein, debunked.

MYTH 1: Eating more protein will lead to kidney damage.

If you are a healthy adult, following the protein recommendations above and increasing the amount based on various individual needs, such as perimenopause or intense exercise, can be done in a healthful way. These recommendations are considered within healthy limits for healthy individuals. However, based on the scientific literature, 1.5 grams per kilogram body weight is a high-protein diet; consuming above the limit of 2.0 grams protein per kilogram body weight can put individuals at risk for developing compromised kidney function, especially when followed long term. High-protein fad diets (think keto, paleo, and Atkins) have been studied, with mixed results regarding potential effects on kidney function, though more research is needed. If you currently have impaired kidney function, are at risk (like people living with diabetes), or are worried, see your healthcare provider or registered dietitian nutritionist (RDN).

MYTH 2: Animal protein is better than plant protein.

These two types of proteins are different, but one is not better than the other. Animal proteins provide all the essential amino acids your body requires, while plant proteins are missing or have less of one or more amino acids. However, plant proteins provide fiber, healthy fats, and other nutrients you don't necessarily find in animal proteins (for example, fiber is only found in plant protein). That is why it is recommended to eat a variety of proteins from both plant *and* animal sources—so you can get the best of both worlds.

MYTH 3: The more protein you eat, the bigger your muscles will get.

Protein and exercise go hand-in-hand, so both are important. However, significantly more protein is not necessarily recommended, as it can also add unnecessary calories and lead to unbalanced meals. For those who lift weights, the recommendation is between 1.2 to 1.7 grams protein per kilogram body weight per day, which should be complemented with weight training.

MYTH 4: You need complementary proteins in one meal.

Plant proteins (like beans, rice, peanut butter, and hummus) do not provide all the essential amino acids needed in one food. It was once believed that combining two plant proteins during a meal (like rice with beans or peanut butter with whole-wheat bread) to complement the amino acids they provide was the best way of taking in plant proteins. This is no longer recommended. Rather, you want to eat a wide variety of plant foods throughout the day and within your long-term healthy eating plan. The combinations of plant-containing-protein foods that you eat throughout the day—which include beans, peas, lentils, nuts, seeds, grains, and vegetables—will provide the variety of amino acids you need.

MYTH 5: **It is impossible to eat too much protein.**

You may have heard that if you eat too much protein, the extra protein simply won't be absorbed. However, your body doesn't work that way. Consuming more protein beyond the daily recommended amount (defined as over 2.0 grams protein per kilogram body weight) can lead to negative consequences. First, you will not be eating a balanced diet; if you eat more protein, you have to eat less carbohydrates and/or fat. This means that you won't be getting some of the nutrients your body needs. In addition, taking in way too much protein can lead to upset stomach, bad breath, excess calories , and possibly poor bone health. In addition, taking in excessive amounts of protein can lead to kidney damage, specifically in those who already have compromised kidneys or are at risk (such as people living with diabetes).

MYTH 6: **You should eat protein before a workout.**

If you're eating a snack an hour before a workout, choose quick-digesting foods like fruit or crackers or modest protein sources such as yogurt. Protein-rich foods are slow-digesting (as explained in "The Science of Protein," in this chapter) and if eaten right before a workout can lead to an upset stomach. To meet your protein needs, eat protein-rich foods during meals and snacks throughout the day, except right before you exercise. If you eat your snack two to three hours before you work out, then it should consist of carbohydrates and moderate protein with less fat.

MYTH 7: **You cannot meet protein needs on a vegan or vegetarian diet.**

When planned properly, you absolutely can get enough protein on a vegan or vegetarian diet. The secret to doing so is including a variety of plant foods that contain protein, including whole grains, beans, peas, lentils, nuts, seeds, and soy products. This makes getting in all your essential amino acids achievable. Plus, those vegan- and vegetarian-based protein foods eaten throughout the day are helpful for keeping you feeling fuller for longer and optimizing workouts—just like animal-based protein foods.

MYTH 8: **You need 1 gram of protein per pound of body weight.**

The recommendation for adults is 0.8 grams protein per kilogram body weight or 0.36 grams protein per pound body weight. Eating 1 gram of protein per pound equates to 2.2 grams per kilogram body weight. As discussed in "How Much Protein Do You Really Need," over 2 grams of protein per kilogram body weight is considered excessive and can leads to kidney damage, specifically in those who already have compromised kidneys or are at risk (such as people living with diabetes).

10 Signs You're Not Getting Enough Protein

Contrary to popular belief, most people in the United States are meeting or even exceeding the recommended amount of protein. However, some situations may lead to inadequate protein consumption—which is considered less than 10 percent of daily calories from protein. This can happen if you are on weight loss medications (such as GLP-1s), which significantly decrease appetite, or if you are on a very restrictive diet. Signs that you're not meeting minimum protein needs include:

FATIGUE AND WEAKNESS.

Not eating enough protein can affect your muscles, especially muscles that help movement. This can certainly happen if you don't meet protein needs as an older adult. Over time, insufficient protein consumption can lead to anemia, which is when your cells don't get enough iron. Protein is needed to make the blood cells that carry oxygen, so you end up feeling tired. Also, not taking in protein when your body needs it can result in losing muscle mass, which can lead to weakness.

MOOD CHANGES.

The building blocks of protein, called amino acids, help make many neurotransmitters in the body, which are chemicals that relay information between cells. If you don't meet minimum protein requirements, then your body can't make enough of these neurotransmitters, which can change how the brain works. For example, if you don't have enough dopamine and serotonin, which are associated with mood and emotion, you can feel depressed, anxious, sad, or irritable. Other factors can also lead to mood changes, so check with your healthcare provider if you are experiencing these symptoms.

HAIR, NAIL, AND SKIN ISSUES.

You need protein to produce elastin, collagen, and keratin, which are all part of your hair, nails, and skin. The end result can be brittle or thinning hair; dry, flaky skin; and fingernails with deep ridges. Other factors can also lead to compromised hair, nail, and skin, so check with your healthcare provider.

DECREASED SLEEP QUALITY.

Protein provides the essential amino acid tryptophan, which is needed to produce serotonin and melatonin. The neurotransmitter serotonin helps promote relaxation, while the hormone melatonin regulates the sleep–wake cycle. As such, if your body doesn't get enough protein, you will not get enough tryptophan to make these sleep-promoting substances, which can lead to disrupted sleep and insomnia.

SWELLING.

Also known as edema, which typically happens in your abdomen, legs, feet, and hands. This is due to the role of protein, which helps manage fluid balance in your body. However, there are other causes of swelling in the body, so always check with your healthcare provider.

There may also be instances when you're not meeting needs for exercise or spacing your protein intake throughout the day during meals and snacks. In these cases, it may result in the following:

DECREASED RECOVERY.

Protein is needed to repair muscle tissue that breaks down during exercise. If you don't take in an appropriate amount of protein throughout the day, this can interfere with rebuilding muscle fibers efficiently, possible prolonged soreness, weakness, and fatigue.

FEELING HUNGRY BETWEEN MEALS.

Taking in protein throughout your day helps slow down how quickly the body is digesting and provides increased satiety. As such, if you aren't taking in moderate sources of protein during meals and snacks, it could lead to feeling hungry between meals.

At this point, you should have a basic understanding of the role of protein in your body and how much protein you need. In the next chapter, I will walk you through various sources of protein, what to look for when buying protein, and the fundamentals of meal prepping so you can take in the protein you need throughout the day.

CHAPTER 2

Building a Protein-Rich Life

Protein sources include both animal and plant, each offering unique nutrients and benefits. Choosing a variety of protein-filled foods throughout the day and week helps ensure you get all the essential amino acids your body needs for muscle maintenance, energy, and overall health. Below is a breakdown of the main animal- and plant-based protein sources and how to include them in a balanced eating plan.

Protein Source Breakdown

Protein sources can come from a combination of animal and plant sources or plants sources alone. Animal sources include poultry, red meat, seafood and fish, eggs, milk and dairy foods. Plant sources include pulses (beans, peas, lentils), nuts and seeds, grains, and vegetables. You can also take in proteins as protein powders, from both animal and plant sources. A breakdown of all the proteins are listed below.

ANIMAL PROTEINS

Poultry: This category includes chicken, turkey, Cornish hen, and duck. Game birds include dove and pheasant. Choose poultry without the skin for less saturated fat. In addition, choose healthy cooking methods such as sautéing, baking, stir-frying, and grilling. Avoid cooking methods like deep-frying.

Red Meat: This category includes beef, veal, pork, lamb, and game such as buffalo, ostrich, rabbit, and venison. Choose lean cuts whenever possible and limit processed red meat like sausages, bacon, and bologna. Minimize sauces high in saturated fat that are made with a lot of butter or cream.

Fish and seafood: The Dietary Guidelines for Americans recommend eating at least 8 ounces of fish per week as part of a healthy eating plan, but to limit fried seafood because it is high in fat and calories. Types of fish to incorporate into your healthy eating plan include fish high in omega-3 fats like salmon, albacore tuna, herring, mackerel, trout, and sardines. Other fish to incorporate include tilapia, flounder, cod, catfish, haddock, orange roughy, and branzino as well as shellfish like clam, crab, shrimp, lobster, scallops, and oysters.

Eggs: According to the American Heart Association, you can include up to 1 whole egg per day as part of a healthy eating plan and balanced with other animal products. The recipes in this cookbook use one large egg as the standard serving.

Milk and dairy foods: Cow's milk and dairy foods like Greek yogurt, cottage cheese, cheese, kefir, and Icelandic yogurt (skyr) all provide protein. If you are lactose intolerant, it is still recommended to choose cow's milk and dairy foods, as many lactose-free, higher-protein options are available. Fortified soy milk provides the closest nutrient profile, including protein, found in cow's milk. Although the Dietary Guidelines for Americans recommends low and nonfat milk as a major part of a healthy eating plan, I've included recipes that use reduced-fat and whole-fat products as well. The key is balancing the types of milk fats as part of a healthy diet.

PLANT PROTEINS

Pulses (also referred to as legumes): The correct term for this protein-filled category is *pulse*, which refers to the dried, edible seeds of legume plants. The United Nations Food and Agriculture Organization recognizes eleven types of pulses; these are the most familiar: dry beans, dry broad beans, dry peas, chickpeas, cow peas, pigeon peas, and lentils. Canned beans, peas, and lentils also fall into this category. When purchasing canned pulses, choose low-sodium, reduced-sodium, or no-added-sodium options. If you purchased regular sodium canned options, rinsing with water before using can reduce up to 40 percent of the sodium.

Nuts and seeds: All nuts and seeds provide protein, healthy fats, fiber, vitamins, and minerals. Some nuts and seeds have slightly higher amounts of protein per serving, including hemp seeds, chia seeds, almonds, peanuts, pistachios, and pumpkin seeds. When choosing nuts and seeds, look for raw or dry-roasted and unsalted.

Grains: Grains contribute some protein as well. The Dietary Guidelines for Americans recommend making half your grains whole. Many whole grains contribute a few grams of protein per serving, but always check the nutrition facts panel for the exact amount. Refined, milled grains also provide a small amount of protein and do contribute to your overall daily protein count. If you choose refined milled grains, make sure they are enriched and fortified. This means they will have a variety of B vitamins, folate, and iron to help close nutrient gaps.

Vegetables: Most vegetables provide some protein. The amount varies depending on the type of vegetable. For example, Brussels sprouts have around 6 grams of protein per cup, while lentils (also considered a vegetable) provide close to 18 grams of protein per cup boiled. While many vegetables are not as high in protein as other sources (such as broccoli, cauliflower, kale, and carrots), they can certainly make contributions and count toward your daily protein intake. Although vegetables do not contain all the essential amino acids you need, by consuming a variety of protein sources throughout the day, you can ensure that you're getting a good mix of amino acids.

ANIMAL PROTEIN POWDERS

Although I recommend a food-first approach to protein, protein powders are another way to add protein to your healthy eating plan. You can find both animal- and plant-derived sources of protein powders. In addition, you can find protein powders that are unflavored and with no added sugars or sweeteners, as well as options in various flavors and with low- or no-calorie sweeteners. Both types are rather pricey, so if you can get enough protein from food every day, you don't need extra powders. Below is an overview of each type of powder available on the market.

Whey protein powder: One of the most popular protein powders is whey protein, which is found in all dairy foods. Cow's milk consists of two proteins: casein and whey. Whey separates from the milk during the cheese-making process. Whey protein is a nutritionally complete protein and releases amino acids, the building blocks of protein, to the muscles quicker than casein. It is also digested rather quickly. In addition, whey is one of the most concentrated sources of leucine, an amino acid responsible for building muscle. This is why research recommends consuming whey protein immediately after an intense workout. I recommend choosing 100 percent whey protein powder, meaning that is the only protein powder found in the container; it is not mixed with any other protein powder. You can find this information listed on the front of the label or read the ingredient list.

Casein protein powder: Casein is derived from cow's milk. Compared to whey, casein has a slower rate of digestion, releasing the amino acids gradually to your muscles. This can be advantageous, as casein protein can help stimulate muscle protein synthesis and improved protein balance during overnight recovery.

Egg-white protein powder: Made from dehydrated egg whites, this protein powder is a complete protein. It is a good option for those looking for dairy alternatives. Most people don't notice any specific taste, and it mixes rather well in beverages.

Collagen protein powder: Collagen powder is made from the animal-rich tissues of cows, pigs, or fish. They provide hydrolyzed collagen peptides, which are small, absorbable pieces of collagen. This protein powder is not complete, meaning it does not provide all the amino acids your body needs in the right amount. Side effects can be digestive issues and lingering taste. Collagen is tasteless and odorless, but the manufacturer may add flavors and sweeteners. It also doesn't change the texture of food, so it can easily be added to beverages, or mixed and blended into smoothies, batters, soups, stews, and more.

PLANT PROTEIN POWDERS

A wide variety of plant-based protein powders are available on the market that are suitable for omnivores, vegetarians, and vegans. You will also find many plant-based protein powder blends. These blends are created for those who believe that they must consume a variety of plant proteins simultaneously to get the full range of amino acids at one time (I debunked this myth in chapter 1; see page 12). Some people may experience gastrointestinal side effects when taking plant-based protein powders, such as gas and bloating. You may need to try a few to see which works best for you. Below is an overview of popular plant-based protein powders and blends.

Soy: Soy protein powder does contain all essential amino acids. You can find soy protein isolate or concentrate. Isolate is made from soybean flakes that have had the fat, carbohydrate, and fiber removed. Concentrate is made from soy flour that had some of the fat and some of the carbs removed. It does have more fiber than isolate.

Bean, pea, or lentil: You can find protein powders made from lentils, from a variety of beans including garbanzo, or from yellow split peas. Peas provide a good amount of all the essential amino acids, while beans and lentils do have limiting amino acids.

Seeds: Although many seeds can be found in protein powder blends, you can find powdered hemp, chia, and flax (some recipes in this cookbook call for these powders). These three seeds also provide omega-3 fats, which give them an added benefit. Seeds are incomplete proteins.

Grains: You can find whole grains like quinoa (technically a seed), amaranth, and millet in protein powders. Many are gluten-free. Some, such as quinoa, provide all the essential amino acids, while most others do not contain all the essential amino acids.

Brown rice: This protein powder is a good choice for people living with food allergies. It is typically gluten-free and has a mild flavor. Brown rice does not contain all the essential amino acids.

Blends: Many plant-based protein powders blend rice, grains, seeds, and beans, peas, or lentils. Blends tend to have added fruit and vegetable powders, sweeteners, and flavors. As mentioned earlier, even if the blend does not contain all essential amino acids, eating a diet that provides a good variety of plant-based proteins will help meet your needs.

Reading Labels & Planning Macros

Food labels can be confusing. My recommendation is to focus on just a few numbers so you don't drive yourself crazy. Below is a rundown of all the information you will find on food labels.

SERVING SIZE

The first thing you should look at on the nutrition facts label is the servings in the package (servings per container) and the serving size. The serving sizes are standardized so you can easily compare similar foods. They are provided in familiar units like cups or tablespoons, followed by the metric amount (usually grams). The serving size reflects the amount people *typically* eat or drink; however, it is not a recommendation of how much you *should* eat or drink.

CALORIES

This provides a measure of the calories in one serving of this food. If the serving size of a food is 1 cup and has 90 calories, and you eat 2 cups, that means you are eating 180 calories.

NUTRIENTS

In the middle of the label, you will find some key nutrients that impact your health. The amount of the nutrients listed refers to the size of the serving. Use the nutrients that help support your individual dietary needs. Look for foods that have more of the nutrients you want to get more of, and less of the nutrients you are trying to limit.

Nutrients to get more of: Dietary fiber, vitamin D, calcium, and potassium are nutrients that most Americans do not get enough of and are considered nutrients of concern that are underconsumed by most of the population.

Nutrients to get less of: Saturated fat, sodium, and added sugars are nutrients listed on the label that may lead to negative health consequences, and Americans tend to overconsume them. This doesn't mean you should have zero of these nutrients, but rather that you should limit them. It is recommended to get no more than 10 percent of total daily calories from saturated fat and added sugar, while the limit on sodium is 2,300 milligrams per day (equivalent to about 1 teaspoon table salt).

ADDED SUGARS VERSUS TOTAL SUGARS

"Added sugars" refers to sugars that are added to the product, such as honey, granulated sugar, or high fructose corn syrup. Those should not be confused with natural sugars found in foods like fruit, milk and dairy, and in starches that are a natural part of the product. Natural sugars, such as honey and maple syrup, become "added sugars" once they are added to a food to give it sweetness. I tend to use my added sugar calories for those. For example, I may add 1 teaspoon honey to my chia seed pudding or 1 teaspoon pure maple syrup to my protein smoothie. Natural and added sugars are combined and listed under *total sugars*, while added sugars are shown separately—that's the number to pay attention to.

PERCENT DAILY VALUES (%DV)

The %DV shows how much a nutrient in a serving of a food contributes to a total daily diet. This helps put the nutrient's numbers, which are found in grams, milligrams, and micrograms, in perspective and on the same scale, which ranges from 0 to 100%DV.

A low source: A %DV of 5 percent or less of a nutrient per serving is considered low.

A good source: A %DV of 10 percent to 19 percent of a nutrient per serving is considered a good source.

An excellent source: A %DV of 20 percent or more of a nutrient per serving is considered a high or excellent source.

According to the National Institutes of Health, it is recommended that adults stay within their calorie limits while choosing food and drinks rich in nutrients. As everyone has individual needs and goals, the guidelines suggest the following for protein, fat, and carbohydrates:

- Carbohydrates: 45 percent to 65 percent of your total calories
- Fats: 20 percent to 35 percent of your total calories
- Protein: 10 percent to 35 percent of your total calories

Specific protein recommendations for adults are 0.8 grams per kilogram body weight, or 0.36 grams per pound body weight. Some individuals need more protein, depending on age, activity level, and health (see page 9). Once you set your protein goals in grams, use the number on food labels (in grams) to add up the total amounts for your meal or snack. Remember, protein intake should be divided throughout the day in meals and snacks, with a target range between 15 to 30 grams at every meal, and no more than 40 grams. Snacks should stay between 10 to 15 grams.

Budget-Friendly Protein Strategies

With food prices on the rise, choosing budget-friendly protein sources can help stretch your food dollar. To determine which proteins offer the best value, the list below uses the recommended daily value of protein along with data from the US Department of Agriculture Thrifty Food Plan Budget, which estimates the cost of a healthy diet for different age and sex groups. The following twenty foods are considered budget-friendly if the cost per serving is 10 cents or less per gram of protein:

Protein	Serving size	Protein *(grams)*	Cost per serving	Cost per gram of protein
Lentils	½ cup	9	$0.15	$0.016
Peanut butter, smooth or crunchy	2 tablespoons	7.6	$0.16	$0.021
Oats	½ cup dry	5	$0.13	$0.026
Plant-based protein powder	1 scoop	25	$0.69	$0.027
Whole-wheat pasta	1 cup	8.8	$0.25	$0.028
Canned tuna	3 ounces	20.1	$0.60	$0.029
Turkey breast	3 ounces	25.6	$0.75	$0.029
Brown rice	1 cup cooked	5.5	$0.17	$0.030
Edamame	1 cup	18.4	$0.63	$0.034
Chicken breast	3 ounces	27.3	$1.03	$0.037
Greek yogurt	7 ounces	19.9	$0.87	$0.043
Cottage cheese	4 ounces	11.8	$0.55	$0.046
Sliced cheese	Per slice	6	$0.28	$0.046
Black beans	½ cup	7	$0.34	$0.048
Chickpeas	½ cup	7	$0.34	$0.048
Kidney beans	½ cup	7.5	$0.40	$0.053
Eggs	1 large chicken egg	6.2	$0.35	$0.056
Quinoa	¾ cup	6	$0.34	$0.056
Tofu	½ cup	10	$0.75	$0.075
Whey protein powder	1 scoop	16.7	$1.18	$0.070

Below are six tips to keep in mind when purchasing protein foods on a budget:

BUY IN BULK.

Purchase larger quantities of non-perishable proteins such as dried beans or dried lentils, or meats, and freeze in individual portions for later use.

PORTIONS MATTER FOR MEATS.

You want to select leaner cuts of meat. Although they may seem more expensive, remember that they have less shrinkage because they are lower in fat. Also, meat portions should be between 3 to 6 ounces, depending on the individual and keeping a little shrinkage in mind during cooking.

CHECK THE FROZEN FOODS AISLE.

Frozen protein sources such as chicken, fish, and seafood tend to be priced lower compared to their fresh counterparts and are just as nutritious. A little secret: Most fish are caught fresh and shipped frozen to major supermarkets throughout the country, but they are just as fresh as the moment they were frozen (which is rather quickly after harvest).

LOOK FOR SALES.

Don't be wary when you find meat on sale at your local market. It is safe and high-quality meat that should be eaten soon after purchase. Check the freshness date on the package or ask the butcher.

MAKE A SPECIFIC GROCERY LIST.

On the list, write down the exact type and amounts of protein you need to buy and stick to it. There is no need to buy more meat than your list calls for.

SHOP AT WAREHOUSE CLUBS.

Warehouse clubs offer big discounts on bulk protein, dairy, meat, chicken, fish, and many other proteins that are fresh, frozen, canned, or shelf-stable (such as nuts and seeds). If you choose to shop at a warehouse club, you will pay less per unit price. However, you do need space to store your food.

Meal Prep Fundamentals

Meal prepping is a technique where you cook and store individual servings of food that can last throughout the week. You can opt to cook just a few recipes to meal prep or you can meal prep most or all of your meals. How much you choose to meal prep is up to you.

There are numerous benefits to meal prepping, which include:

Saving money: This is especially helpful with pricier foods such as meat and seafood, where you purchase the exact amount you need for the recipe and pack the amount in each individual container.

Saving time: Spending time over the weekend or over one or two evenings a week can save time that you would otherwise spend prepping on a busy weeknight. This allows you more time on those early mornings or late nights where you want to work out or spend quality time with your family.

Eating healthier: Having planned meals throughout the week can help minimize those app food orders or stopping by the closest fast-food joint in desperation.

Controlling weight: To help meet your weight loss, weight maintenance, or even bulking goals, keeping portions and protein amounts in check within meals and snacks can be a hurdle. By boxing meals and snacks, you'll be using a great tool for portion control.

FIVE STEPS TO MEAL PREPPING

When meal prepping, I recommend following these five steps:

Step 1: Choose when to meal prep. Select one or two days a week to meal prep. Most people like to prep one day over the weekend, but you can also choose to prep on another day during the week that works best for you. You can also split up your meal prepping over two shorter days as opposed to doing everything at once. Do whatever works best for you.

Step 2: Decide which meals to meal prep. This cookbook tags recipes that are appropriate for meal prepping and provides storage, reheating, and serving instructions for all meal-prepped recipes. When choosing which recipes to meal prep, decide how many recipes to start with. If you are new to meal prepping, start with only a few recipes. If you feel that you can handle more, then go for it!

When selecting recipes, choose a variety of protein sources so you can get different proteins and nutrients from the ingredients used. Remember, when meal prepping, you should choose a recipe that can be refrigerated for up to four days—so you will eat each portion for a meal four days in a row (unless you freeze it). This helps minimize how many dishes you cook up at one time. In addition, keep in mind that you want meals balanced with protein (plant or animal), grains (especially whole grains), veggies, fruit, milk and dairy products, and healthy fat.

Step 3: Go food shopping. My secret to food shopping is to make a list based on the flow of the supermarket—and I like to do it with a pen and paper (I know, I am old-school!). However you choose to write your shopping list, if you organize it by types of foods it helps prevent those last-minute dashes through the supermarket because you forgot one food back in aisle 1. I organize my list with the following categories: fruits and vegetables, meat/poultry/fish, pantry items, frozen aisle, and milk/dairy foods.

I also recommend creating your list from your kitchen. This way as you go through the ingredients of each recipe you can check your pantry, refrigerator, and freezer for the ingredient. This helps minimize buying an ingredient you already have and helps keep your food spending in check.

Step 4: Prep and cook. Meal prepping is about efficiency and saving time. When you meal prep numerous recipes, use the following tips to organize what to prep and cook when.

- Read through all the recipes before you begin.
- Prep ingredients for recipes that take longer to cook. For example, chop onions and marinade meats.
- Begin longer cooking recipes, especially those that will be baked in the oven or cooked stovetop for over 20 minutes. While these dishes are cooking, you can prep other recipes.
- Leave shorter recipes for down time. For example, dressings and simple snack recipes can be prepped when other recipes are cooking.

- Cook the remaining recipes, which you should be able to assemble in a flash since you have already prepped most of the ingredients.
- Portion and pack meals and snacks into single-serve containers. Store extra meals in the freezer, when applicable.

Step 5: Portion, pack, and store. If you want to ensure you're getting the amount of protein listed in the recipe and to keep calories in check (especially if you are trying to lose or maintain weight), then make sure to portion your recipe and store in single-serve containers. This makes it easy to heat and eat without any fuss.

Smart Protein Swaps

With so many protein-filled ingredients on store shelves, you can easily add a few grams of protein to any meal or snack by swapping in certain ingredients or adding others to your dish. You can use either ingredient, but if you're trying to add a bit more protein to your meal or snack, the following foods can help you meet your individual needs. This is especially important with vegan and vegetarian meals, where it's tougher to meet your target range in meals and snacks and those few extra grams of protein can help.

Remember, more isn't better when it comes to protein. Spread your protein throughout the day, with a target range between 15 to 30 grams at every meal, and no more than 40 grams at every meal. Aim for between 10 to 15 grams of protein for snacks. The following page includes easy swaps you can make for ingredients that have more protein compared to its counterpart.

SIMPLE PROTEIN SUBSTITUTIONS

Instead of...	Use...
Traditional yogurt	Greek yogurt or skyr
Traditional milk	Ultra-filtered milk (about 13 grams protein per cup)
Sour cream	Greek yogurt, or blended cottage cheese
Cream cheese	Cottage cheese, or replace half the cream cheese with blended cottage cheese
Traditional pasta	High-protein pasta like chickpea or lentil, or pastas labeled as "high protein"
All-purpose flour	High-protein flour In baked goods, replace up to one-third of the flour with unflavored protein powder like whey, soy, chickpea, or oats
White rice	Quinoa, amaranth, teff, farro, spelt
Mayonnaise	In pasta or chicken salad, replace up to half with Greek yogurt As a condiment for sandwiches, use hummus
Butter or jam on toast	Nut butter like peanut or almond butter
Croutons or small crackers for soups and salads	Nuts, seeds, or roasted chickpeas
Lettuce	Kale or spinach

Easy Tips to Incorporate Protein

If you're looking to add a few grams of protein to dishes, here are a few tips and tricks that you can use. If you're trying to get the most out of plant-based proteins, the goal is to take in a variety of proteins so you can get all those amino acids throughout the day. You can find some of these included in the recipes of this cookbook.

FLAX, HEMP, OR CHIA SEEDS

Add ground seeds to casseroles, batters, sauces, and marinades. Use whole seeds for salads or to sprinkle over sweet snacks and desserts.

NUTS AND SEEDS

Sprinkle on salads or oatmeal.

PEANUT OR ALMOND BUTTER POWDER

Add to smoothies, shakes, and batters (such as pancakes and muffins) to add flavor and protein.

CHEESE

Sprinkle on omelets, pasta dishes, salads, or soups.

NUTRITIONAL YEAST

Sprinkle this vegan alternative to cheese anywhere you would cheese, like popcorn, pasta, and potato dishes.

FROZEN EDAMAME OR PEAS

These both have more protein compared to other frozen vegetable counterparts (such as carrots or corn). Add to soups, pasta dishes, stews, and stir fries.

NUT BUTTERS

Add to smoothies, oatmeal, sauces, batters, and spreads and use to dip apples, pears, and celery.

WHOLE GRAINS LIKE BROWN RICE, FARRO, AND QUINOA

Add to soups, salads, and stews.

OATS AND OATMEAL

Add to liquid (like milk) and let stand 10 minutes before adding other ingredients to smoothies, shakes, and smoothie bowls. Cook oatmeal in milk or soymilk, and once it is cooked and in a bowl, add a splash more milk or soymilk to add more protein before serving.

EGG

Add to your snack and sprinkle with everything bagel seasoning.

CHICKPEAS OR BEANS

Add to your salads or side dishes (like beans to your grains).

CHAPTER 3

Cooking and Planning for Protein Success

Mastering Protein Cooking Techniques

Whether plant- or animal-based, include protein at every meal and snack to meet your daily protein targets. Since no one wants rubbery chicken or overcooked steak, the guide below lists popular proteins and provides tips for perfectly cooking each one. If you don't perfectly cook a protein the first time, just remember that practice makes perfect. All the cooking methods included are healthy options (the only method to minimize is deep-frying). From achieving perfectly flaky fish to tender, juicy chicken, this cooking guide has you covered.

ANIMAL PROTEIN COOKING METHODS

Poultry

Below are the best cooking methods for chicken and turkey.

Cooking	More Information	Best For
Braising	Results in juiciness and flavor This technique slow cooks chicken in a small amount of liquid, resulting in flavorful stews and casseroles	Whole chicken Drumsticks Thighs
Grilling	Results in a smoky flavor and nice, tasty char Can use an outdoor grill during warm weather or a grill pan for indoor grilling	Thighs Drumsticks Breasts
Sautéing	Quick stovetop method using a hot pan with a small amount of fat (like oil or butter) to cook chicken Versatile for different seasonings	Breasts Thighs
Poaching	When you cook chicken in a simmering liquid Results in juiciness and flavor, as this method helps retain moisture and keeps the meat tender and juicy	Breasts Thighs

Cooking	More Information	Best For
Roasting	Roasting in the oven cooks the chicken with dry heat Results in a juicy, tender, and often crispy chicken	Whole chicken Drumsticks Thighs

Beef

Below are the best cooking methods for beef. Note that the names of cuts of beef vary throughout the country. A good resource to find the various names for cuts of beef is www.BeefItsWhatsForDinner.com.

Cooking	More Information	Best For
Braising	A moist-heat cooking method This method browns the meat and then cooks it covered in a small amount of liquid at a low temperature for an extended period	Tougher cuts of beef like: Cross rib roast Chuck tender roast Blade chuck roast Top blade Brisket Beef short ribs
Pan-searing	Quick stovetop method using a hot pan with a small amount of fat Is a dry-heat method Results in a golden-brown crust on tender cuts like filet mignon using high heat in a skillet	Thick-cut, boneless steaks that are 1 to 1.5 inches thick: Ribeye New York strip Filet mignon (tenderloin) Sirloin
Roasting	Uses dry heat to cook larger cuts of meat in a closed oven Results in a juicy, tender beef	Ribeye roast Bottom round roast Shoulder petite tender Eye of round roast

Cooking	More Information	Best For
Grilling	Results in a smoky flavor and nice, tasty char on tender cuts Can use an outdoor grill during warm weather or a grill pan for indoor grilling	Many cuts do well on the grill, such as: Boneless strip steak Boneless and bone-in ribeye steak Porterhouse/T-bone steak Flat iron steak Tenderloin steak (filet mignon) Top sirloin steak Bottom round steak Eye of round steak Kabobs (skewers) Ground beef patties Shoulder steak
Skillet-to-oven	Start by searing a steak in a skillet and then finish by cooking in a low-heat oven, providing even cooking for thick cuts This is a combination cooking method	Cowboy steak Flat iron steak Shoulder petite tender medallions New York strip Ribeye Porterhouse or T-bone Sirloin Filet mignon
Stewing	Meat is completely submerged in liquid; ideal for less-expensive cuts This is a moist-heat cooking method	Stew meat
Stir-frying	Quickly cooks thin strips of beef in a hot pan or wok This quick dry-heat cooking method keeps the meat tender	Flank steak Inside skirt steak Ranch steak Denver steak

Pork

Below are the best methods for cooking pork:

Cooking	More Information	Best For
Braising	For tougher cuts Start by browning the meat, then cooking it slowly in a covered pot with a small amount of liquid This method breaks down connective tissues, yielding tender, flavorful meat	Shoulder Ham
Grilling	Ideal for smaller to medium cuts Impart a smoky flavor Can use an outdoor grill during warm weather or a grill pan for indoor grilling	Chops Tenderloin Medallions
Roasting	For tender cuts of meat Simple method Uses dry-heat cooking For extra flavor, sear for extra flavor before placing in the oven to finish	Chops Tenderloin Medallions
Searing/pan-frying/sautéing	For tender cuts of pork Uses high heat to create a flavorful, golden-brown crust on the pork's surface This can be the first step before finishing in the oven	Chops Tenderloin Medallions
Stewing	Cook meat in a larger amount of liquid so the meat is completely submerged until it becomes tender For tougher cuts	Shoulder Ham

Fish and shellfish

Below are the best methods for cooking fish and shellfish:

Cooking	More Information	Best For
Braising	Uses moist-heat cooking Slowly cooks fish and shellfish in liquid, typically with vegetables, to tenderize it	Firm-fleshed varieties that can hold their shape in liquid without falling apart (such as cod, monkfish, or black cod) Shellfish such as mussels
Broiling	Uses dry-heat cooking Creates a browned crust	Firm-fleshed fish such as salmon, tuna, swordfish, halibut, and mahi-mahi Shellfish such as shrimp, scallops, clams, mussels, and lobster (tails)
Grilling	Uses dry-heat cooking Quick cooking method Adds flavor Can use an outdoor grill during warm weather or a grill pan for indoor grilling	Firm, oily fish such as salmon, tuna, swordfish, and mahi-mahi Shellfish such as shrimp, scallops, oysters, and lobster Whole fish
Pan-searing (pan-frying)	Uses dry-heat cooking This method cooks in a hot pan with oil to create a crispy exterior while inside remains moist and tender	Firm white fish such as cod, halibut, snapper, and bass Meaty fish such as salmon and tuna Shellfish such as shrimp and scallops

Cooking	More Information	Best For
Poaching	Uses moist-heat cooking Gently cooks fish in a simmering liquid such as water, broth, or stock without drying it	Lean white fish such as cod, flounder, halibut, and snapper Fatty fish such as salmon, tuna, and trout Shellfish such as shrimp, scallops, clams, mussels, and various crabs and lobsters
Roasting	Simple method Uses dry-heat cooking Roast fish in a preheated oven set to 400°F to 450°F for about 10 minutes per inch of thickness. A whole fish may take slightly longer (about 10-12 minutes per 8 ounces at 350°F, or 15-20 minutes at 400°F).	Fatty fish such as salmon and tuna Firmer, flaky white fish such as halibut, cod, and snapper Shellfish such as scallops and clams Thicker fillets Whole fish Fish steaks
Steaming	Uses moist-heat cooking Gently cooks fish, preserving its delicate flavor and texture	Mild, flaky white fish such as cod, sole, and sea bass Delicate fish such as halibut Shellfish such as clams (littlenecks, steamers), mussels, and shrimp
Stewing	Build a flavorful broth base first, and then add the fish or seafood late in the cooking process to prevent overcooking Fish and seafood cook very quickly, about 3-10 minutes	Fish chunks like cod, halibut, or snapper Seafood like shrimp, scallops, mussels, clams

PLANT PROTEIN COOKING METHODS

Below you will find common plant proteins and the best ways to cook them to maximize flavor and texture.

Food	More Information	Cooking Method(s)
Beans (dried or canned)	Dried bean varieties require soaking and cooking Soaking in water with flavorings like herbs, onions, or bay leaves adds more flavor Soaking reduces cooking time, improves texture, and makes them easier to digest by removing some complex sugars that can cause gas Canned beans and peas can be purchased as low-sodium, reduced-sodium, and no added sodium Rinsing canned beans and peas reduces the sodium by up to 40 percent	Wet-heat methods such as: Simmering Boiling
Edamame	Typically found frozen shelled and in-shell Can be blended or mashed for spreads or dips	Boiling Steaming Sautéing Microwaving
Lentils	No soaking required Flavor with herbs, onions, and pepper during cooking Season with salt after cooking to help preserve their texture	Simmering

Food	More Information	Cooking Method(s)
Peas (whole, split, frozen, canned)	Whole pea varieties require soaking and cooking; split peas do not Best to cook for a short amount of time over high heat	Frozen peas: Sautéing Microwaving Frozen or fresh peas: Steaming Stir-frying
Tempeh	First steam or simmer to remove any bitterness, then add a marinade, and then cook using your preferred method	Baking Pan-frying
Texturized vegetable protein (TVP)	Typically requires rehydration in water or broth in a microwave-safe bowl with plastic wrap	Once rehydrated, cook in sauté pan on the stove top with a bit of oil
Tofu	Includes extra-firm, firm, and silken varieties Press firm or extra-firm to remove water Recommend marinating to add flavor To hold up shape, use extra-firm Typically cut into 1-inch pieces	Baking Pan-frying/sautéing Stir-frying Air frying Grilling Braising

Common Cooking Mistakes

When you head into the kitchen, you want to get every step right so you end up with the most flavorful protein meal. But mistakes happen. Below you'll find seven common cooking mistakes when it comes to protein foods.

***MISTAKE #1:* Overcrowding the pan.**

When you fill the pan with too much protein at one time, it lowers the temperature and results in steaming the food, which becomes soggy instead of browned.

Fix It: Cook your protein foods in batches to ensure that each piece has enough space in the pan to sear correctly.

***MISTAKE #2:* Not patting seafood dry.**

When the surface on seafood such as fish or shrimp is moist, it will prevent it from getting a good sear, which can result in a mushy texture.

Fix It: Pat your fish and seafood dry with a single-use paper towel before cooking. Discard paper towel after using.

***MISTAKE #3:* Not marinating lean meat.**

Lean cuts of meat such as chicken breasts or pork loin can get dry if you don't marinate them.

Fix It: Marinate your lean meat for at least twenty minutes or up to twenty-four hours to add moisture, flavor, and help keep it tender.

***MISTAKE #4:* Overcooking shrimp.**

Shrimp cooks incredibly quickly, and cooking it too long can result in a rubbery texture.

Fix It: Shrimp typically needs to cook two to four minutes per side. Visually, cook until they form a gentle C shape and are opaque.

***MISTAKE #5:* Cooking eggs on too low of a heat.**

If you cook eggs on a very low heat, they can end up sticking to the pan.

Fix It: Cook eggs on medium-high heat, which prevents sticking.

***MISTAKE #6:* Adding salt or acidic ingredients too early when cooking lentils.**

If you add salt or an acidic ingredient such as citrus juice or vinegar too early, it can result in tough lentils.

Fix It: For tender lentils, add salt at the end of the cooking process (or after it's cooked) and wait toward the end of cooking to add the acidic ingredients.

MISTAKE #7: Not allowing the poultry or meat to rest before slicing.

If you cut poultry or meat too early without resting, all the flavors pour out onto the cutting board, resulting in less flavor and tenderness. It also results in soggy skin (like for chicken).

Fix It: Allow poultry and meat to rest for five to twenty minutes (depending on size) before slicing. Letting the meat rest allows the juices to redistribute back into the protein, leaving you with a more tender and juicy protein.

Protein Cooking Temperature Guide

Whether you are cooking plant- or animal-based proteins, the only way to tell if your food is cooked through is by using a thermometer. Having a food thermometer on hand allows you to check the internal temperature. Below you will find the different types of food thermometers available and the recommended minimum internal cooking temperatures for common protein foods.

TYPES OF THERMOMETERS

There are several types of thermometers to choose from. The first type is the one I have in my home and recommend using when cooking plant- and animal-protein dishes, including the recipes in this cookbook. Remember to store your thermometer in an easily accessible location, as you should be using it every time you cook. Using a thermometer doesn't only allow for meeting food safety guidelines, but it also yields a more consistent and better-quality product than cooking by time alone. Visual cues are not recommended to tell the doneness of your proteins, especially animal-based proteins.

Instant-read thermometers: These thermometers are inserted 2 to 2-½ inches into the thickest part of the food (or diagonal when checking temperatures of thinner dishes like egg dishes or burgers). This thermometer reads the internal cooking temperatures typically in ten to twenty seconds.

Thermometer forks: This combination is perfect for grilling and can read the temperature in two to ten seconds. To measure the temperature, insert the fork at least ¼ inch deep in the thickest part of the food, and ensure that the sensor in the fork is fully inserted.

Meat thermometer: Similar to instant-read thermometers, analog meat thermometers have a larger dial, which makes them easier to read. A meat thermometer is inserted into a joint of meat or whole turkey or chicken and stays there throughout the roasting process. To check the temperature, just check the dial. You can also find digital versions that can be programmed to beep when your desired temperature is met.

MINIMUM INTERNAL COOKING TEMPERATURES

Most foods have a recommended minimum internal cooking temperature. Don't count out cooked plant-based foods, as handling them or not cooking them properly can potentially lead to foodborne illness; having said that, most have a lower overall risk. As long as you follow the instructions for cooking plant dishes, the risk of foodborne illness is at a minimum. As such, only higher-risk protein foods are listed below. Some seafood, due to their thinness, do not have a specific internal cooking temperature. Visual signs of doneness are provided in the chart below for those foods.

Food	Minimum Internal Cooking Temperature
Beef, pork, veal, and lamb: steaks, chops, and roasts	145°F and allow to rest for at least 3 minutes
Ground meats and sausages	160°F
Ground poultry	165°F
Ham: fresh or smoked (uncooked)	145°F and allow to rest for at least 3 minutes
Fully cooked ham (to reheat)	Reheat cooked hams packaged in USDA-inspected plants to 140°F and all others to 165°F
All poultry: breasts, whole bird, drumsticks, thighs, wings, ground poultry, giblets, and stuffing	165°F

Food	Minimum Internal Cooking Temperature
Eggs	160°F
Fish: whole of fillet (salmon, tuna, tilapia, pollock, bass, cod, catfish, trout)	145°F or flesh is opaque and separates easily with fork
Rabbit or venison (wild or farm-raised)	160°F
Shrimp, lobster, and crabs	Flesh pearly and opaque
Clams, oysters, and mussels	Shells open during cooking
Scallops	Flesh is milky white or opaque and firm
Tofu	165°F
Casseroles (meat and meatless)	165°F
Plant-based burgers (such as a bean burger)	160°F
Leftovers (animal or plant)	165°F

Flavor Strategies for High-Protein Foods

Classic French cooking often flavors foods with butter, salt, and sugar. Consuming too much of these ingredients has been linked to an increased risk of chronic disease such as obesity, type 2 diabetes, and cardiovascular disease. These flavor enhancers are best minimized, as most people already consume more than enough. Fortunately, there are many ways to add flavor to both animal- and plant-based proteins. You'll find nine ideas below.

JUICES

One hundred-percent fruit and vegetable juices provide natural sugars and a fruity flavor that helps balance earthy flavors from plant-based protein powders, such as pea or hemp in smoothies and shakes. They can also add a depth of flavor to pork, chicken, and beef. Get creative by using pomegranate, tart cherry, pineapple, orange, grape, carrot, and tomato juice.

VINEGAR

Vinegar has a light, tangy taste and activates your taste buds without the addition of many calories or fats. When tenderizing, vinegar (an acidic ingredient) breaks down the protein structure, which makes meat softer and allows the seasoning to penetrate deeper. This adds depth and complexity to protein-based dishes. Choose from a variety of vinegars, such as balsamic, apple cider, rice, white, red or white wine, or vinegars infused with herbs or other flavors.

STOCKS AND BROTHS

Stocks, broth, and bone broth are made with vegetables and herbs to create a rich, savory flavor that complements dishes such as stews and braised food. Use them to add flavor to chicken thighs or in a sauce for turkey and chicken.

RUBS AND MARINADES

There are dry and wet rubs. Dry rubs are a powdery mix of herbs, spices, and other seasonings, while a wet rub or paste contains a small amount of wet ingredients, such as mustard. Both dry and wet rubs can be used on meats immediately before cooking to enhance flavor.

Marinades are liquids used before cooking to add flavor, moisten food, and tenderize meats. They contain an acidic ingredient, such as wine, citrus juice, or vinegar. Poultry and meat should be marinated for at least twenty minutes or up to twenty-four hours. Fish, shellfish, and tofu should marinate for at least twenty minutes but no longer than about two hours so they don't fall apart.

AROMATIC VEGETABLES

This group of vegetables—which includes onions, scallions, leeks, shallots, and chives—adds distinct flavors and aromas to both plant and animal proteins. Many protein dishes start by sautéing onion and garlic in a bit of oil to add those unbelievable flavors and depth to dishes like vegetarian or beef chili.

WINE, BEER, AND SPIRITS

Wine, brandy, cognac, liqueurs, and beer can add flavor without many calories. The longer these alcoholic beverages are cooked, the more their calories and alcohol content are reduced. When cooking animal protein dishes, adding alcohol helps in a variety of ways, including tenderizing and adding a complexity of flavors. In addition, the acidity of wine can cut through the richness of a fatty meal, which helps balance the final flavors. Finally, compounds in red wine can interact with proteins, enhancing both color and aroma in sauces for steaks and stews.

COULIS

A coulis is a sauce made from a purée of vegetables and/or fruit. The tangy, acidic flavor of coulis helps cut through the richness of protein. For example, a cherry or cranberry coulis can stand up to the savory flavors of pork, lamb, or duck. Coulis also adds flavor and moisture to leaner meats, such as pork tenderloin and boneless, skinless chicken breast.

SALSA

Salsas add a complex mix of flavors when paired with chicken or fish. Chunky salsas can also contribute texture. A variety of salsa can be used, including traditional tomato, pineapple, corn, or salsa verde.

CHUTNEY

A chutney is a chunky sauce made with fruits, vegetables, and/or herbs. Chutneys can be served as a condiment alongside meat, used as a glaze, or incorporated into marinades and sauces. For example, chicken and turkey pair well with cranberry, apple, or mango chutney. Pork pairs well with apple or pear chutney, while steak or roast beef pair well with a tomato chutney.

Meat Prep Mastery

Try the following techniques for tender, flavorful meat every time.

POUND CHICKEN.

Chicken cooks best when you pound it to an even thickness, typically for chicken breasts unless they are thin sliced. For traditional chicken breasts, cover them in plastic wrap to prevent splattering and pound the thicker end with a mallet. This promotes even cooking and tenderizes the chicken by breaking down muscle fibers.

MARINATE.

Marinating helps add flavor and helps tenderize. For best results, marinate poultry and meat for at least twenty minutes or up to 24 hours. Tofu, fish, and shellfish should be marinated for at least twenty minutes or up to 2 hours.

BRING POULTRY AND MEAT TO ROOM TEMPERATURE.

Cooking cold poultry or meat can dry out the exterior. Remove it from the refrigerator for twenty minutes before cooking. Avoid leaving it out longer, as pathogenic microorganisms can grow on raw protein at room temperature, especially when left out for over two hours (or over one hour when the temperature is 90°F or above).

PAT DRY.

Surface moisture on whole chicken, skin-on chicken, meat, fish, and shellfish prevents browning. To achieve a crispy texture, use a single-use paper towel to thoroughly pat them dry. Discard the paper towel and wash your hands when done.

DO NOT OVERCOOK.

Use your thermometer to ensure proteins reach the minimum internal cooking temperature without overcooking. This applies to poultry, meat, fish and shellfish, eggs, and tofu.

COVER LOOSELY WITH FOIL TO REST.

Small cuts like chicken thighs and breasts should rest for five to ten minutes, while larger roasts should rest for fifteen to thirty minutes.

Slice against the grain for the most tender poultry, meat, and fish.

Strategic Meal Planning System

When planning your protein-filled meals for the week, it is important to come up with a system that will make your life a whole lot easier. Below are three sections to review each time before building your meal plan. At first, meal planning will take a bit longer, but once you get into the swing of things it should become increasingly easier.

1. Make Goal-Specific Adjustments

Before starting your meal plan, pre-determine the amount of protein (in grams) that you will aim for per day. Use the chart below (and see page 8, "How Much Protein Do You Really Need") to set your daily protein goals. Your protein needs can change with weight fluctuations, aging, and changes in your activity level. That's why it's important to calculate your protein requirements regularly or review your numbers to see if any adjustments are needed.

Who Are You?	What Is Your Goal?	To Calculate Protein Needs Use...
Healthy adult men and women age nineteen and above who are not very physically active	Weight loss Weight maintenance	0.8 grams per kilogram body weight OR 0.36 grams per pound body weight
Perimenopausal woman who is sedentary or works out once or twice a week Man between forty to sixty years of age who is sedentary or works out once or twice a week	Weight loss Weight maintenance Restore muscle mass	1.0 to 1.2 grams per kilo-gram body weight OR 0.45 to 0.54 grams per pound body weight Calculate toward the upper limit if you are more active

Who Are You?	What Is Your Goal?	To Calculate Protein Needs Use...
Healthy adult man or woman who is nineteen years or older, who works out sixty to ninety minutes most days of the week Perimenopausal woman who works out sixty to ninety minutes most days of the week	Weight loss Weight maintenance Restore muscle mass Build muscle Support muscle repair Muscle recovery	1.2 to 1.6 grams of protein per kilogram body weight OR 0.54 to 0.72 grams per pound body weight
Adult man or woman who lifts weights or is training for a running or cycling event five to seven days per week	Support muscle repair Build muscle Muscle recovery	1.2 to 1.7 grams per kilogram body weight OR 0.54 to 0.77 grams per pound body weight

2. Weekly Planning Template

Use the following template to plan your weekly meals. Most people need one to three snacks per day, in the morning, afternoon, and/or evening, respectively. Snack if you go four or five hours between meals or if you find yourself so hungry between meals that you need to eat. Choose how many snacks you need and when you will eat them. Remember to calculate protein from your entire plate, and not only your protein dish. Sides like grains and vegetables, and beverages like milk and soymilk, also contribute to protein needs. You don't need to be 100 percent exact on your protein goal—if you are a gram or two higher or lower, that is close enough.

Week of:_______________ Total grams of protein per day: _______________

	Breakfast	Lunch	Dinner	Snack 1	Snack 2	Snack 3	Total
Sunday	Meal protein total = ____ grams	Meal protein total = ____ grams	Meal protein total = ____ grams	Meal protein total = ____ grams	Meal protein total = ____ grams	Meal protein total = ____ grams	Daily protein total = ____grams
Monday	Meal protein total = ____ grams	Meal protein total = ____ grams	Meal protein total = ____ grams	Meal protein total = ____ grams	Meal protein total = ____ grams	Meal protein total = ____ grams	Daily protein total = ____grams
Tuesday	Meal protein total = ____ grams	Meal protein total = ____ grams	Meal protein total = ____ grams	Meal protein total = ____ grams	Meal protein total = ____ grams	Meal protein total = ____ grams	Daily protein total = ____grams
Wednesday	Meal protein total = ____ grams	Meal protein total = ____ grams	Meal protein total = ____ grams	Meal protein total = ____ grams	Meal protein total = ____ grams	Meal protein total = ____ grams	Daily protein total = ____grams
Thursday	Meal protein total = ____ grams	Meal protein total = ____ grams	Meal protein total = ____ grams	Meal protein total = ____ grams	Meal protein total = ____ grams	Meal protein total = ____ grams	Daily protein total = ____grams
Friday	Meal protein total = ____ grams	Meal protein total = ____ grams	Meal protein total = ____ grams	Meal protein total = ____ grams	Meal protein total = ____ grams	Meal protein total = ____ grams	Daily protein total = ____grams
Saturday	Meal protein total = ____ grams	Meal protein total = ____ grams	Meal protein total = ____ grams	Meal protein total = ____ grams	Meal protein total = ____ grams	Meal protein total = ____ grams	Daily protein total = ____grams

If you're not used to tracking anything in your meal plan, I recommend starting with protein grams only. You can then choose to add calories, and then the other macros: carbs and fat. Do whatever is best for you. Tracking apps can make tracking easier.

3. Balancing Protein on Your Plate

A healthy plate is balanced with protein, fats, and carbs. You can build and balance your plate in two ways: visually or by crunching the numbers. If you don't like to sit and calculate everything, then the visual method is for you. This will allow you to balance your plate with various food groups and get a variety of nutrients. Be mindful of the grams of protein in both meals and snacks. You can also "crunch the numbers" and simply do the math. If you want to know exactly how many grams of every macro and/or your total daily calories, use this method.

The Visual Method. Start by filling half your plate with vegetables and/or fruit. Next, fill one-quarter of your plate with lean meats and protein foods such as skinless chicken breast, beans, or tofu. Last, fill the final quarter of your plate with starches such as brown rice, quinoa, pasta, or potatoes. Complement your plate with some healthy fat, such as avocado or a serving of vinaigrette dressing, and about 1 cup from the dairy group (aim for 3 cups per day). Don't forget to opt for a low- or no-calorie drink like water, unsweetened iced tea, or sparkling water.

Use this formula to build your plate:

- **Fruits and vegetables:** 50 percent
- **Starches and starchy vegetables:** 25 percent
- **Proteins:** 25 percent (lean animal proteins, such as skinless chicken breast, pork tenderloin, fish, and eggs, or plant proteins like beans, peas, lentils, nuts, tofu)

Complement with:

- **Healthy fat:** a small portion of healthy fat (two slices of avocado, four to five olives, or one to two tablespoons of vinaigrette)

- **Dairy group:** 1 cup of the dairy group is equivalent to 1 cup of milk, yogurt, or soymilk or 1½ ounces of natural cheese
- **Low or no-calorie beverage:** To meet daily fluid needs, complement meals with low- or no-calorie beverages, such as water, sparkling water, unsweetened iced tea

Crunch the Numbers. If you want to know your total calories and macros (protein, fat, and carbs) for the day, use this method. This book walks you through the calculations to determine the percentage of calories from protein and also provides guidance so you can calculate all your macros on your own.

To calculate the percent calories from protein:

1. Calculate how much protein you need based on your weight (see page 49).
2. Determine your calorie needs by using an online calculator, which uses your gender, age, height, weight, and activity level to calculate your dietary reference intake (DRI). Either search online for "dietary reference intake" or you can find it on the US Department of Agriculture's website: www.nal.usda.gov/human-nutrition-and-food-safety/dri-calculator.
3. Calculate the calories from protein you should eat by multiplying your grams of protein by 4 calories per gram. For example, if your daily protein intake is 70 grams, multiply 70 × 4 to get 280 calories from protein.
4. You can then divide 280 calories by your total daily calories and multiply that result by 100 to determine the percentage of your daily total calories you should be getting from protein.

For example, for 70 grams of protein on an 1,800 calorie diet, it would be calculated as:

70 grams protein × 4 calories per gram of protein = 280 calories from protein

(280 calories from protein/1,800 calorie diet) × 100 = 15.5 percent calories from protein

To calculate the remaining macros:

To calculate the grams of carbs and fats you need, use the following recommendations. Crunching the numbers is very tedious, so as long as you get around the percentage listed below, you are good to go:

- **Carbohydrates:** 45 percent to 65 percent of your total calories
- **Fats:** 20 percent to 35 percent of your total calories
- **Protein:** 10 percent to 35 percent of your total calories

You will need this information to help you calculate:

- **Carbohydrates:** 4 calories per gram
- **Fats:** 9 calories per gram
- **Protein:** 4 calories per gram

Seasonal Considerations

Eating seasonally mostly applies to fruits and vegetables that are available at your local markets. The more variety of fruits and vegetables that you take in, the wider range of nutrients you'll be feeding your body. Plus, buying fruits and vegetables that are in season can help keep your food dollar on budget.

Each recipe in this cookbook has a *Toby's Tip*, where I oftentimes recommend easy swaps, especially with produce. You are always welcome to make those swaps to meet your individual needs. If you find a produce swap at your local farmers' market you think would work well in a dish, then go for it!

SALAD PROTEIN BOOSTERS

Love salads, but want to boost the protein? Check out these easy salad additions that can up your protein in any salad:

Food Group	Food	Portion	Protein *(grams)*
Seeds	Hemp hearts	1 tablespoon	3
	Chia seeds	1 tablespoon	3
	Flax seeds	1 tablespoon	2
	Pumpkin seeds	1 tablespoon	1
	Sunflower seeds	1 tablespoon	2

Food Group	Food	Portion	Protein *(grams)*
Nuts	Peanuts (dry roasted)	2 tablespoons	4
	Almonds (dry roasted)	2 tablespoons	4
	Walnuts (halves)	2 tablespoons	2
	Pine nuts	2 tablespoons	2
	Pistachios (dry roasted)	2 tablespoons	3
Cheese	Feta (crumbled)	2 tablespoons	3
	Goat cheese (crumbled)	1 ounce	4 to 6 (depending on brand)
	Part-skim mozzarella (shredded)	2 tablespoons	4
	Parmesan (grated)	2 tablespoons	4
	Reduced-fat cheddar (shredded)	2 tablespoons	4
Vegan cheese alternative	Nutritional yeast	2 tablespoons	5
Beans, peas, lentils	Chickpeas (canned)	½ cup	5
	Black beans (canned)	½ cup	6
	Lentils (cooked)	½ cup	9
	Edamame (shelled and cooked)	½ cup	8
	Cannellini beans (canned)	½ cup	8
	Kidney beans (canned)	½ cup	8
	Green peas (frozen)	½ cup	4

Food Group	Food	Portion	Protein *(grams)*
Quick proteins	Rotisserie chicken (skinless)	3 ounces	24
	Hard-boiled egg	1 large	6
	Grilled chicken (leftovers)	3 ounces	26
	Canned sardines (packed in water)	4.4 ounce can (can sizes vary)	25
	Canned chicken breast (packed in water)	3 ounces (drained)	15
	Canned chunk light tuna (packed in water)	3 ounces (drained)	20
	Canned salmon (packed in water)	3 ounces (drained)	18

Batch Cooking & Prep Strategies

When you're trying to meet your daily goal of protein within a balanced meal, batch cooking various protein, starch, and vegetable and/or fruit options is a smart way to be prepared. This helps save money on cooked convenience proteins or other foods you may end up picking up last minute at the local market or restaurant.

Below you'll find information to help you batch cook various proteins, what to look for in storage containers, best cooling and storage techniques, how to reheat proteins, and time-saving prep tips. You'll also find simple tips to keep your batch-cooked proteins safe to eat.

BATCH COOKING METHODS

There are two primary ways to prepare batch-cooked meals.

Meal prepping: When you prep the entire balanced meal and store individual portions to eat during the week (see page 27). The meal plans at the end of this chapter use this method.

Ingredient batch cooking: Preparing individual components of the plate, such as grilled chicken, sautéed tofu, steamed broccoli, roasted Brussels sprouts, baked potato, and cooked farro, which are then combined into different balanced meals throughout the week.

The following table lists several easy ways to ingredient batch cook popular proteins.

Food	Recommended Cooking Instructions	Cook Time	Minimum Internal Cooking Temperature
Grilled chicken breast (boneless, skinless)	Season both sides with salt and pepper (or season as desired). Heat grill pan or grill and coat with olive oil or nonstick cooking spray.	6 to 8 minutes, flipping once, or until it reaches its minimum internal cooking temperature	165°F
Sautéed chicken breast (boneless, skinless)	Season both sides with salt and pepper (or season as desired). Heat sauté pan on medium with 1 to 2 tablespoons olive oil.	6 to 8 minutes, flipping once, or until it reaches its minimum internal cooking temperature	165°F
Stovetop ground lean beef (at least 90 percent lean)	Preheat large skillet over medium-high heat with 1 to 2 tablespoons olive oil. Add the ground beef and break it up as it cooks. Season before or during cooking, and after make any adjustments to your liking.	8 to 10 minutes, or until it reaches its minimum internal cooking temperature	160°F

Food	Recommended Cooking Instructions	Cook Time	Minimum Internal Cooking Temperature
Sautéed boneless pork chop	Season both sides with salt and pepper (or season as desired). Heat large skillet with 1 to 2 tablespoons olive oil.	3 to 4 minutes on each side, or until it reaches its minimum internal cooking temperature	145°F
Roasted salmon fillets	Preheat oven to 425°F and coat a baking dish with non-stick cooking spray. Season with salt and pepper (or season as desired).	10 to 15 minutes, depending on the thickness, or until reaches the proper minimum internal cooking temperature	145°F
Hard-boiled eggs	Place eggs in a medium saucepan and cover with cold water. Place the saucepan over high heat and bring to a boil; cook for 3 minutes. Remove saucepan from the heat, cover, and let stand 15 minutes. Drain and run cold water over the eggs until completely cool, about 10 minutes. Once cooled, peel the eggs.	Cook 3 minutes; let stand in covered pot for 15 minutes; cool completely for 10 minutes	Cook until yolk and whites are firm

Food	Recommended Cooking Instructions	Cook Time	Minimum Internal Cooking Temperature
Sautéed Extra-Firm Tofu	Drain water from the tofu container. Wrap tofu in paper towels or a clean dish towel, and place on clean plate or cutting board. Place a heavy skillet or pan on top to apply pressure, allowing it to press for at least 30 minutes. Cut the tofu into 1-inch cubes. Season both sides with salt and pepper (or marinate and allow to sit in the refrigerator covered for 20 minutes to 2 hours). Heat sauté pan on medium with 1 to 2 tablespoons olive oil.	4 to 5 minutes, flipping until golden brown on all sides	Until golden brown
Boiled canned chickpeas	Rinse and drain chickpeas. Add chickpeas to a medium saucepan with ½ cup water per can, with salt and pepper, and desired seasoning. Bring mixture to a boil over high heat.	Once boiling, reduce heat to medium and simmer for 5 minutes before draining	Until chickpeas are soft and tender (do not overcook)

Food	Recommended Cooking Instructions	Cook Time	Minimum Internal Cooking Temperature
Boiled dried lentils	Place the dried lentils in a fine-mesh sieve and rinse under cold running water; remove any small pebbles or debris. In a medium saucepan combine every 1 cup of dried lentils with 2 to 3 cups water or broth. Bring to a boil over high heat. Once boiling, reduce the heat to low and simmer, uncovered. Drain. Season with salt and pepper, or seasoning of choice.	20 to 30 minutes, uncovered, or until reaches desired tenderness (cook time varies by lentil type)	Until desired tenderness

SELECTING STORAGE CONTAINERS

For meal prepping and batch cooking, storage containers are essential. Airtight containers help maintain the flavor, texture, and color of stored foods. Having the correct containers helps reduce exposure to air, which also helps maintain the food's quality and makes it last longer and taste fresher throughout the week.

When selecting storage containers, keep in mind the following:

Single or multiple compartments. Do you like your foods touching in one compartment or are you a "my foods can't touch" kind of person? This is a personal decision. When batch cooking, however, you do want deeper containers so you can store a few days' worth of the food (like grilled chicken breasts or hard-boiled eggs).

Stackable/nestable. Maximize the space in your cabinets by containers that use space wisely. Choose containers that can fold or stack nicely when not in use, so your cabinets stay organized.

BPA-free. The industrial chemical bisphenol A (BPA) has been around since the 1960s, but now many people feel most comfortable purchasing BPA-free food storage containers. Although the US Food and Drug Administration (FDA) found that BPA is safe in small amounts, for frequent use look for the BPA-free label indicated on the package. Also, purchase containers that are made to use with food, as opposed to containers that are meant to store non-food items (such as office supplies). Those types of containers may contain BPA and are not food-safe. Glass containers are a good option and do not contain BPA.

Leakproof. Read the online reviews about the containers you are considering buying. The worst is when you purchase a nice set of containers only to find out they keep leaking all over everything!

Microwave-, dishwasher-, and freezer-safe. Some of the meals will be cooked, cooled, and then stored in the freezer; when you're ready to eat them, they will be thawed and reheated in the microwave. It is easiest to do this in one dish rather than transfer them all the time. As such, I recommend finding containers that have all of these characteristics listed on the label.

COOLING FOOD PROPERLY

Place cooked food in shallow containers and allow to come to room temperature (about 70°F). This should take no longer than twenty to thirty minutes. Once the food reaches 70°F, refrigerate promptly to allow to completely cool. Do not leave cooked food to cool for more than two hours at room temperature after cooking or more than one hour if the temperature is 90°F or above. To help the food cool quicker, divide the food into smaller portions and transfer to shallow containers. This is much quicker than leaving the food in large quantities (like a big pot of stew) to cool. Store foods in an airtight container to help keep the bacteria and other pathogens out and retain moisture.

STORING FOOD PROPERLY

Once food is cooled properly, leftovers can be stored in the refrigerator for three to four days or frozen for three to four months. I like to use frozen leftovers within two months so I don't forget about them. Also, if you store leftovers too long in the freezer they can lose moisture and flavor.

Before storing food, don't forget to label it with the contents and the date it was stored. This will help you keep better track of how long your food has been stored and hopefully allow for better rotation of what you store.

REHEATING FOOD PROPERLY

There are several ways you can reheat your food. Using the microwave is quick and easy, but just remember that heat is distributed unevenly. Be sure to stir food halfway through reheating. After cooking food to reach a minimum internal temperature of 165°F, let it stand for two minutes to allow the heat to distribute evenly.

Alternatively, you can use your stove top or oven to reheat the food to a minimum internal cooking temperature of 165°F.

Food can be reheated more than once, as long as it was handled properly from preparation through cooking, cooling, and reheating.

SEVEN TIME-SAVING BATCH COOKING PREP TIPS

Batch cooking will certainly save you time throughout your busy workweek. But you can save even more batch-cooking time by following the tips below:

1. **Plan ahead.** Before you begin, decide how much food and how many meals you want to prep for the week. Then create a shopping list and plan out your meals for the week.

2. **Choose versatile foods.** Opt for foods and recipes that you can easily pair or use in multiple ways. For example, sautéed tofu can be used as a main dish with cooked brown rice and steamed broccoli, or you can top a green vegetable salad with tofu. Also, opt for recipes that you can cook once and use twice or thrice. For example, chili can be eaten in a bowl, in quesadillas, and over tortilla chips to make protein-filled nachos.

3. **Prepare your tools.** Before starting your prep, make sure your tools are clean, you can find the lids to your containers, you have your thermometer handy, and you have everything needed on the counter. This will keep everything accessible so you don't spend extra time looking for a tool.

4. Prepare ingredients. Chop, slice, dice, mince, measure, and do any other prep you need to do for each recipe. This helps save time—especially when you have multiple dishes cooking at once.

5. Make double or triple portions. You may choose to make double or triple portions to store in the freezer for another busy week.

6. Label and date. Every container should be labeled and dated to ensure that you know what is in each container and that you use the food on time.

7. Choose storage locations. You can portion your food and opt to store them in the fridge for use during this week, or store in the freezer for another time. Most foods will keep in the refrigerator for up to four days or in the freezer for up to two months (follow the recommendations in the recipes).

TEN FOOD SAFETY DOS AND DON'TS

1. Do wash your hands often. Wash your hands before you begin cooking, after a bathroom break, after taking out the garbage, after handling raw meat, and any other time you contaminate them.

2. Do have a meat thermometer on hand. The only way to tell if your food, including meat, fish, and poultry, is cooked through is to use a meat thermometer. You can find the best meat thermometer for you on page 44.

3. Do separate raw and cooked food. Cross-contamination occurs when bacteria or other microorganisms from raw food are transferred to the ready-to-eat or cooked food. Keep raw and cooked or ready-to-eat food (like fruit) separate, and use separate cutting boards for each food. If you only have one cutting board, be sure to wash and sanitize it before using it with different foods. Don't forget to wash and sanitize any knives and utensils you reuse as well.

4. Do wash your reusable grocery bags regularly. Juices of food and other forms of contamination can get into your reusable grocery bags. Wash them between each use. Once they are overused, toss them.

5. Do keep hot food hot and cold food cold. Keep cooked food warm by loosely covering it after being cooked. Cold food should remain in the refrigerator until you're ready to serve it. This helps minimize growth of pathogenic microorganisms.

6. Don't let cooled food sit out. Divide the cooked food into its individual containers, and once it hits 70°F then store them in the refrigerator or freezer immediately. The cooked food should not sit out for over two hours (or over one hour if the temperature is 90°F or above).

7. Don't thaw meat on the counter. When you thaw meat on the counter, pathogenic bacteria can divide to such high amounts that it can make you sick, even if you cook the food properly. The juices of the meat can also contaminate your countertop and even drip into drawers and make a huge mess. Meat, fish, and poultry can be thawed several ways. You can thaw food in the refrigerator overnight; larger pieces of meat (like a ham or whole turkey) may take a few days. You can thaw by running smaller pieces of meat, poultry, or fish under cool, running water. If you leave it in a bowl in the sink, change the water every thirty minutes. You can also thaw in the microwave, but the food should then be cooked immediately after using any cooking method you choose.

8. Don't wash food with soap or detergents. Never wash foods, including fruits, vegetables, and meat, using soap, bleach, detergents, or anything else not made for food. It ends up in the food that you are eating and can potentially make you sick. It can also ruin the quality of the food.

9. Don't store raw meat, chicken, and fish in the upper shelves of the refrigerator. This can lead to another form of cross-contamination, where the raw foods can drip onto other cooked or ready-to-eat foods. Not only can it potentially make you sick, but it will also make a mess in your refrigerator.

10. Don't rinse raw meat, poultry, and fish in the sink. The splatters of the water can contaminate your kitchen sink and counters. It is not recommended to rinse your meat, poultry, and fish before preparing and cooking.

PROTEIN STORAGE QUICK REFERENCE

Storage times for foods can vary. Below is a quick guide to storing protein safely.

Food	Type	Refrigerator *(40°F or below)*	Freezer *(0°F or below)*
Luncheon meat	Opened package or deli sliced	3 to 5 days	1 to 2 months
Luncheon meat	Unopened package	2 weeks	1 to 2 months
Bacon	—	1 week	1 to 2 months
Sausage	Fully cooked from chicken, turkey, pork, or beef	1 week	1 to 2 months
Sausage	Purchased frozen	After cooking, 3 to 4 days	1 to 2 months
Hamburger, ground meats, and ground poultry	Hamburger, ground beef, turkey, chicken, other poultry, veal, pork, lamb, and mixtures of them	1 to 2 days	3 to 4 months
Fresh beef, veal, lamb, and pork	Steaks, chops, and roasts	3 to 5 days	4 to 12 months
Ham	Fresh, uncured, cooked or uncooked	3 to 5 days	3 to 4 months
Fresh poultry	Chicken or turkey, whole	1 to 2 days	1 year
Fresh poultry	Chicken or turkey, pieces	1 to 2 days	9 months
Fin Fish	Fatty fish (bluefish, catfish, mackerel, mullet, salmon, tuna, etc.)	1 to 3 days	2 to 3 months
Fin Fish	Lean fish (cod, flounder, haddock, halibut, sole, etc.)	1 to 3 days	6 to 8 days

Food	Type	Refrigerator *(40°F or below)*	Freezer *(0°F or below)*
Fin Fish	Lean fish (pollock, ocean perch, rock-fish, sea trout)	1 to 3 days	4 to 8 days
Shellfish	Live clams, mussels, oysters, and scallops	5 to 10 days	Not recommended
Shellfish	Shrimp, crayfish	3 to 5 days	6 to 18 Months
Eggs	Raw eggs, in shell	3 to 5 weeks	Do not freeze in shell; beat yolks and whites together, then freeze
Eggs	Raw egg whites and yolks, out of shell Note: Yolks do not freeze well	2 to 4 days	12 months
Eggs	Hard-boiled eggs	1 week	Do not freeze
Eggs	Casseroles with eggs	After baking, 3 to 4 days	After baking, 2 to 3 months
Soups and stews	Vegetable or meat added	3 to 4 days	2 to 3 months
Leftovers	Cooked meat and poultry	3 to 4 days	2 to 6 months
Leftovers	Chicken nuggets or patties	3 to 4 days	1 to 3 months
Leftovers	Pizza	3 to 4 days	1 to 2 months
Leftovers	Cooked plant foods, including beans and tofu	3 to 4 days	2 to 6 months

Quick-Assembly Meals

Once you batch cook your foods, the next step is to create a satisfying meal that helps meet your mealtime protein needs. Because you have already prepared all the meal components, there is no need for cooking. Now it's all about adding some flavor and assembly. Below are my simple steps for quick-assembly meals.

CREATE A PLATE.

When assembling meals, fill half your plate with vegetables and/or fruit, one-quarter with protein, and the last one-quarter with grains or starchy vegetables (like potatoes). If your meal has animal protein (meat, poultry, fish, or shellfish), then a cooked portion of 3 to 6 ounces (depending on your protein needs) will meet your meal goals. If you're following a vegetarian diet, then you may need to add some additional protein sources to your meal by sprinkling your salad with chia seeds, sprinkling cheese over your cooked vegetables, or adding Greek or Icelandic (skyr) yogurt for dessert.

PAY ATTENTION TO PORTIONS.

If you follow the basic formula above, you should not only have a balanced plate but you'll also get the protein grams you need. If you have higher calorie needs, then use a 9-inch dinner plate. If you have lower calorie needs, then use a 7-inch dinner plate. This will also help manage portion sizes easily.

ADD SPICES AND OTHER FLAVORS.

If you have batch-prepared food such as grilled chicken or sautéed salmon, you can enjoy it plain, but these foods do taste better when flavorings are added. Spices are a good way to add flavor for few calories and no saturated fat or added sugar. You can purchase Italian seasoning or blends like "fish seasoning" or "chicken seasoning"—just check the label for sodium if that is of concern. Refer to "Flavor Strategies for High-Protein Foods" on page 45 for more ideas.

15-Minute Meal Formula

Using the Quick Assembly Meals template (page 67), here are several combinations you can easily put together with dishes you have batch-prepared:

BOWL

About 1 to 1½ cups grain or starchy vegetable like potatoes; 3 to 6 ounces of cooked protein or ¾ to 1 cup of beans, peas, lentils; and at least 1 cup of cooked vegetables. Sprinkle with flavoring of choice. For vegetarian meals, sprinkle with nutritional yeast, shredded cheese, seeds, or nuts for some added protein.

SALAD

A vegetable base of 1 to 2 cups of vegetables; 3 to 6 ounces of cooked protein or ¾ to 1 cup of beans, peas, lentils; and at least 1 cup of cooked vegetables. Drizzle with vinaigrette or other dressing of choice (minimize use of creamy high-saturated fat dressings). Top with croutons or crushed tortilla chips, or serve with a small roll or whole-wheat bread. For vegetarian meals, sprinkle with nutritional yeast, shredded cheese, seeds, or nuts for some added protein.

SANDWICH OR WRAP

Fill the sandwich or wrap with about 2 ounces of protein; about ½ cup smashed beans, peas, and lentils or 1 to 2 ounces of cheese; add vegetables such as lettuce, kale, and cucumbers; and flavor with hummus, pesto, or other condiments that contain healthy fat or protein. Serve with a side of vegetables (green salad, raw vegetables, or cooked vegetables).

Strategic Snacking for Protein Goals

Snacks are mini meals that should help fill nutrient gaps between meals. It's a perfect opportunity to insert protein, which can help you meet your individual protein goals and help you stay satisfied between meals. It also means you don't *only* want to eat protein during your snack—combining it with one or two other food groups provides an array of nutrients your body needs.

A good target is between 10 to 15 grams of protein and 150-300 calories per snack, depending on your individual protein and calorie goals.

The timing of snacks also matters. If you go four to five hours between meals or you are feeling very hungry between meals or during a certain time of day, that is a good time to insert a snack. Having protein with that snack can help curb hunger so you can get to your next meal without feeling super hungry and grabbing whatever food you find quickly as a result. Adding fiber and some healthy fat to that snack can also add satiety.

If you regularly work out, weight train, or train for a big race, what you choose to snack on differs. Usually you want snacks that contain fiber and protein to slow digestion, but when you exercise, the recommendations change depending on timing.

What you eat before you work out is based on the timing of your meal or snack. You also need to consider how well you tolerate or digest certain foods, and if that food choice is a good option for you. The table that follows can help you determine what to eat before exercise based on your individual eating schedule. Many of the options for 3 hours or less are portable, so you can pre-pack them or stock up and grab-and-go.

Timing	Types of Food	Examples
4 hours before	A balanced meal with carbohydrates, protein, and fat	Oatmeal made with ultra-filtered milk and topped with berries and chopped nuts Turkey and cheese sandwich with tomato soup Sautéed salmon with baked potato and a green salad
2 to 3 hours before	Carbohydrates and moderate protein with less fat	Greek yogurt or Icelandic (skyr) topped with granola Trail mix made with dried fruit and nuts Energy bar Half a peanut butter and jelly sandwich Hummus with pita chips
1 hour or less before	Easily digestible carbohydrates	Smoothie Pretzels Fruit like watermelon, banana, apple, pear Granola bar Half a bagel with jam Drinkable yogurt

Post-exercise, you should eat both protein and carbohydrates to help promote recovery and build muscle. If you eat protein on its own, your body won't reap all the benefits. A rule of thumb post-moderate- to high-intensive exercise is to aim for a protein-to-carbohydrate ratio of 1:3, which is 1 gram of protein for every 3 grams of carbohydrates. For endurance athletes, a protein-to-carbohydrate ratio of 1:4 is often used. However, your ideal post-workout snack really depends on your activity, duration, and fitness level. For example, riding an indoor bike for twenty minutes at moderate speed doesn't warrant the same post-workout snack as attending a HIIT workout or an hour spin class. The meal or snack should also include antioxidant-filled foods that help fight inflammation. For maximum recovery, eat your post-exercise snack or meal immediately after your workout (ideally no later than forty-five minutes after).

Also remember to hydrate before, during, and after exercise. If you exercise for more than one hour of moderate activity, then electrolyte sports drinks are a good idea.

5 Prep-Ahead Snack Strategies

1. Pre-portion trail mix for 1 week.
2. Keep drinkable yogurts in your refrigerator.
3. Make protein balls or bites (see page 261) on Sunday and store in the refrigerator.
4. Prepare hummus and crackers or pretzels and store in the refrigerator.
5. Stock up on granola bars at home or in your work desk.

Your Five-Day Protein Meal Prep Meal Plans

Here you will find four different meal-prepping meal plans for busy workweeks. As described earlier, meal prepping is about preparing and cooking several meals over one or two days and eating those meals throughout the week. The recipes typically make between four to six servings, so you eat four or so during the week and freeze the rest for a busy week down the line. It also means that you're typically eating the same lunch or dinner most days of the week. This also helps save time when meal prepping (so you don't prepare fifteen different meals for the week) and saves money too. The meal plans go from Monday through

Friday, with a bit of extra food you can either enjoy over the weekend or freeze for another week.

The four meal plans below include:

- **Meal plan 1:** An 1,800-calorie meal plan for a perimenopausal woman who is an omnivore and works out several days a week.
- **Meal plan 2:** A 1,900-calorie meal plan for a post-menopausal woman who is a vegetarian and works out several days a week.
- **Meal plan 3:** A 2,550-calorie meal plan for an adult man who is an omnivore and works out most days of the week.
- **Meal plan 4:** A 2,000-calorie meal plan for an adult woman who is an omnivore and works out most days of the week.

Use the meal plan that closest suits your needs and tweak whatever you need to individualize it. Happy, healthy meal prepping!

Meal Plan 1

For: Perimenopausal woman
Weight: 150 pounds
Exercise: 45 minutes, 3 to 4 days a week

Calories: 1,800
Protein needs: 1.3g/kg body weight = **89 grams per day**
Diet: Omnivore

	Monday–Thursday	Friday
Breakfast	**Blueberry-Lemon Chia Seed Pudding** *Total Calories: 317* *Carbohydrates: 33g* *Protein: 18g* *Fat: 14g*	**Peaches and Cream Milkshake** *Total Calories: 373* *Carbohydrates: 66g* *Protein: 20g* *Fat: 6g*
Morning Snack	**Chocolate Protein Balls** *Total Calories: 290 Carbohydrates: 36g Protein: 9g Fat: 14g*	

	Monday–Thursday	Friday
Lunch	**Three-Bean Plant-Forward Chili** **1 small dinner roll** **1 teaspoon unsalted butter** *Total Calories: 517* *Carbohydrates: 72g* *Protein: 28g* *Fat: 16g*	**Sheet Pan Spicy Tofu and Vegetables** **1 small dinner roll** **1 medium apple** *Total Calories: 589* *Carbohydrates: 80g* *Protein: 23g* *Fat: 24g*
Afternoon Snack	**Layered Chocolate-Raspberry Popsicles** *Total Calories: 56 Carbohydrates: 6g Protein: 6g Fat: 1g*	
Dinner	**Ground Pork Stir-Fry with Mushroom, Zucchini, and Carrots** **1 cup cubed cantaloupe** *Total Calories: 544* *Carbohydrates: 63g* *Protein: 30g* *Fat: 20g*	**Skillet Ground Beef with Sweet Potatoes** **Lemon-Garlic Spinach** **1 cup sliced strawberries** *Total Calories: 568* *Carbohydrates: 39g* *Protein: 33g* *Fat: 32g*
Nutrition Information	*Total Calories: 1,798* *Carbohydrates: 209g* *Protein: 92g* *Fat: 66g* *Carbohydrates: 46.5%* *Protein: 20.5%* *Fat: 33%*	*Total Calories: 1775* *Carbohydrates: 212g* *Protein: 90g* *Fat: 63g* *Carbohydrates: 48%* *Protein: 20%* *Fat: 32%*

MEAL PLAN 1: RECIPES

- Three-Bean Plant-Forward Chili (page 173)
- Blueberry-Lemon Chia Seed Pudding (page 120)
- Chocolate Protein Balls (page 271)
- Ground Pork Stir-Fry with Mushroom, Zucchini, and Carrots (page 242)
- Layered Chocolate-Raspberry Popsicles (page 280)
- Lemon-Garlic Spinach (page 251)
- Peaches and Cream Milkshake (page 104)
- Sheet Pan Spicy Tofu and Vegetables (page 158)
- Skillet Ground Beef with Sweet Potatoes (page 220)
- Spicy Black Bean Dip (page 263)

MEAL PLAN 1: SHOPPING LIST

PANTRY

- Almonds, raw
- Beans, low-sodium black (2 × 15.5-ounce can)
- Beans, low-sodium kidney (2 × 15.5-ounce can)
- Beans, low-sodium pinto (1 × 15.5-ounce can)
- Black pepper, ground
- Broth, low-sodium chicken
- Broth, low-sodium vegetable
- Cayenne pepper
- Chia seeds
- Chia seeds, ground
- Chilies, diced green (1 × 4-ounce can)
- Chili powder
- Chili powder, chipotle
- Chocolate chips, semi-sweet
- Cocoa, unsweetened
- Coriander, ground
- Coriander seeds
- Cornstarch
- Cumin, ground
- Dates, Medjool
- Flour, all-purpose
- Ginger, ground
- Hemp seeds
- Hemp seeds, ground
- Honey, liquid
- Juice, pomegranate or cranberry
- Nutritional yeast
- Oats, rolled
- Oil, extra-virgin olive
- Oil, olive
- Oil, sesame
- Oregano, ground
- Paprika, ground
- Paprika, smoked
- Parsley, dried
- Peanut butter, creamy
- Peanut butter powder
- Peanuts, unsalted
- Peppers, roasted red
- Roll, small dinner (4)
- Quinoa
- Rice, brown basmati
- Rice vinegar, unseasoned
- Salt, kosher
- Soy sauce, reduced sodium
- Tomatoes, low-sodium fire-roasted diced (2 × 14.5-ounce can)
- Tomato paste (1 × 6-ounce can)
- Vanilla extract, pure
- Whey protein isolate

FRUIT, VEGETABLES, HERBS & SPICES

- Apple (1)
- Blueberries
- Broccoli florets (2 cups)
- Cantaloupe
- Carrots, baby
- Carrots
- Celery
- Garlic, bulb (3)
- Lemon (2)
- Lime (1)
- Mushrooms, Portobello (1 × 6-ounce package)
- Onion, red (1)
- Onion, yellow (2)
- Pepper, jalapeño (2)
- Pepper, red bell (2)
- Spinach, baby (1 × 1-pound package)
- Strawberries
- Sweet potato (3)
- Zucchini (1)

PROTEIN

- Beef, ground, at least 90 percent lean (1 pound)
- Pork, ground, at least 90 percent lean (1 pound)
- Tofu, extra-firm (1 × 1-pound package)

DAIRY

- Cheese, cheddar, reduced fat
- Cheese, Mexican, reduced fat, shredded
- Cheese, ricotta
- Milk, ultra-filtered skim (1 × 52-ounce bottle)
- Yogurt, Greek, nonfat vanilla (1 cup)
- Yogurt, Greek, reduced fat, plain (1 cup)
- Yogurt, Icelandic or skyr (½ cup)

FROZEN

- Peaches, frozen sliced
- Raspberries

MEAL PLAN 1: STEP-BY-STEP PREP

1. Prepare the **Sheet Pan Spicy Tofu and Vegetables** through step 2 (page 158).
2. While the tofu is being pressed, prepare the **Layered Chocolate-Raspberry Popsicles** through step 2 (page 280).
3. Continue making the **Sheet Pan Spicy Tofu and Vegetables,** steps 3 to 5 (page 158).
4. Continue making the **Layered Chocolate-Raspberry Popsicles,** steps 3 to 4 (page 280).
5. Pack the **Sheet Pan Spicy Tofu and Vegetables** for the freezer to be eaten on Friday, step 7 (page 158).
6. Prepare the **Ground Pork Stir-Fry with Mushroom, Zucchini, and Carrots** (page 242).
7. Prepare the **Three-Bean Plant-Forward Chili,** steps 1 to 2 (page 173).
8. Pack the **Three-Bean Plant-Forward Chili,** step 4 (page 173).
9. Prepare the **Skillet Ground Beef with Sweet Potatoes,** steps 1 to 3 (page 220).
10. Prepare the **Blueberry-Lemon Chia Seed Pudding** (page 120).
11. Pack the **Skillet Ground Beef with Sweet Potatoes** for the freezer to be eaten on Friday, step 5 (page 220).
12. Prepare the **Lemon-Garlic Spinach** (page 251).

13. Prepare the **Chocolate Protein Balls** (page 271).
14. Prepare the **Peaches and Cream Milkshake** (page 104) right before eating and prepare the **Spicy Black Bean Dip** (page 263) during the week, as it only lasts for 4 days in the refrigerator.

Meal Plan 2

For: Post-menopausal woman
Weight: 150 pounds
Calories: 1,900
Exercise: 45 minutes, 3 to 4 days a week
Protein needs: 1.4g/kg body weight = **95 grams per day**
Diet: Vegetarian (eats eggs and dairy foods)

	Monday-Thursday	Friday
Breakfast	**Apple-Walnut Cottage Cheese Bowls** *Total Calories: 285* *Carbohydrates: 23g* *Protein: 17g* *Fat: 15g*	**PB & Raspberry Shake** *Total Calories: 278* *Carbohydrates: 37g* *Protein: 26g* *Fat: 2g*
Morning Snack	**Chocolate Protein Balls** *Total Calories: 290* *Carbohydrates: 36g* *Protein: 9g* *Fat: 14g*	**Banana Walnut Protein Bread** *Total Calories: 327* *Carbohydrates: 35g* *Protein: 9g* *Fat: 18g*
Lunch	**Sheet Pan Eggs with Chickpeas and Vegetables** *Total Calories: 407* *Carbohydrates: 49g* *Protein: 20g* *Fat: 16g*	**Smashed Chickpea Dill Sandwich** **Tajin Baked Red Potatoes** *Total Calories: 574* *Carbohydrates: 76g* *Protein: 25g* *Fat: 23g*
Afternoon Snack	**Spicy Black Bean Dip** *Total Calories: 127* *Carbohydrates: 22g* *Protein: 8g* *Fat: 1g*	**Pecan Pie Yogurt Bowl** *Total Calories: 261* *Carbohydrates: 20g* *Protein: 12g* *Fat: 15g*

	Monday - Thursday	Friday
Dinner	**Lentil Stew** **1 small dinner roll** **Panna Cotta with Strawberry-Chia Sauce** *Total Calories: 735* *Carbohydrates: 118g* *Protein: 41g* *Fat: 16g*	**Quinoa and Kale Bowls with Poached Egg** **1 clementine** *Total Calories: 439* *Carbohydrates: 57g* *Protein: 22g* *Fat: 16g*
Nutrition Information	*Total Calories: 1930* *Carbohydrates: 248g* *Protein: 95g* *Fat: 62g* *Carbohydrates: 51%* *Protein: 20%* *Fat: 29%*	*Total Calories: 1892* *Carbohydrates: 225g* *Protein: 94g* *Fat: 74g* *Carbohydrates: 47%* *Protein: 17%* *Fat: 35%*

MEAL PLAN 2: RECIPES

- Apple-Walnut Cottage Cheese Bowls (page 119)
- Banana Walnut Protein Bread (page 267)
- Chocolate Protein Balls (page 271)
- Lentil Stew (page 156)
- Panna Cotta with Strawberry-Chia Sauce (page 276)
- PB & Raspberry Shake (page 100)
- Pecan Pie Yogurt Bowl (page 270)
- Quinoa and Kale Bowls with Poached Egg (page 170)
- Sheet Pan Eggs with Chickpeas and Vegetables (page 166)
- Smashed Chickpea Dill Sandwich (page 141)
- Spicy Black Bean Dip (page 263)
- Tajin Baked Red Potatoes (page 257)

MEAL PLAN 2: SHOPPING LIST

PANTRY

- Baking powder
- Bay leaves
- Beans, low-sodium black (1 × 14.5-ounce can)
- Beans, low-sodium Great Northern or cannellini beans (1 × 14.5-ounce can)
- Black pepper, ground
- Bread, multigrain (8 slices)
- Broth, low-sodium vegetable
- Capers
- Chia seeds
- Chickpeas, low-sodium (2 × 15.5-ounce can)

- Chocolate chips, semi-sweet
- Cinnamon, ground
- Cocoa, unsweetened
- Cooking spray, nonstick
- Coriander seed, ground
- Cumin, ground
- Dates, pitted
- Flaxseed, ground
- Gelatin powder
- Hemp seeds, ground
- Honey, liquid
- Lentils (2 × 15.5-ounce cans)
- Maple syrup, pure
- Mustard, Dijon
- Nutritional yeast
- Oats, rolled
- Oil, avocado
- Oil, extra-virgin olive
- Oil, olive
- Oregano, dried
- Paprika, smoked
- Peanut butter, smooth
- Peanut butter powder
- Peanuts, unsalted
- Pecans, dry-roasted, unsalted
- Pita, whole-wheat (large)
- Quinoa
- Red pepper flakes
- Red peppers, roasted
- Rolls, small (4)
- Salt
- Salt, kosher
- Sesame seeds, dry-roasted, unsalted
- Sugar, granulated
- Sunflower seeds, dry-roasted
- Tahini
- Tajin seasoning
- Thyme, ground
- Tomatoes, crushed (1 × 15-ounce can)
- Vanilla extract, pure
- Vinegar, apple cider
- Walnuts, raw
- Whey protein isolate powder, unsweetened
- Za'atar seasoning

FRUIT, VEGETABLES, HERBS & SPICES

- Apple, Honeycrisp, Cosmic Crisp, Granny Smith, or Fuji (2)
- Banana, medium (3)
- Carrots, baby
- Carrots
- Celery
- Clementine (1)
- Dill
- Garlic, bulb (1)
- Kale (7 cups)
- Lemon (3)
- Lettuce, romaine
- Lime (1)
- Mushrooms, button (1 × 10-ounce container)
- Onion, red (1)
- Onion, yellow, medium (1)
- Parsley, flat-leaf
- Pepper, green bell
- Pepper, jalapeño (1)
- Potatoes, red (7 medium)
- Potatoes, russet (2 medium)
- Scallions
- Shallot (1)
- Spinach, baby
- Strawberries
- Tomato, cherry
- Tomato, plum (5)

PROTEIN

- Eggs, large (8)

DAIRY

- Butter, unsalted
- Cheese, crumbled feta
- Cheese, reduced fat Swiss (4 slices)
- Cottage cheese, 2 percent
- Milk, ultra-filtered (1 × 52-ounce bottle)
- Whipping cream, heavy
- Yogurt, Greek, nonfat plain (2 cups)
- Yogurt, Greek, nonfat vanilla (½ cup)
- Yogurt, Greek, reduced fat (2 percent) plain

FROZEN

- Peas
- Raspberries

MEAL PLAN 2: STEP-BY-STEP PREP

1. Prepare the **Sheet Pan Eggs with Chickpeas with Vegetables,** steps 1 to 6 (page 166).
2. While the sheet pan recipe is cooling, prepare the **Apple-Walnut Cottage Cheese Bowls** (page 119).
3. Pack the **Sheet Pan Eggs with Chickpeas with Vegetables,** step 8 (page 166).
4. Prepare the **Lentil Stew,** steps 1 to 2 (page 156).
5. Prepare the **Banana Walnut Protein Bread** (page 267).
6. While the **Banana Walnut Protein Bread** is cooking, pack the **Lentil Stew,** step 4 (page 156) and prepare the **Chocolate Protein Balls** (page 271).
7. Prepare the **Panna Cotta with Strawberry-Chia Sauce,** steps 1 to 5 (page 276).
8. Prepare the **Quinoa and Kale Bowls with Poached Egg** (page 170).
9. Prepare the **Spicy Black Bean Dip** (page 263).
10. Pack the **Panna Cotta with Strawberry-Chia Sauce,** step 7 (page 276).
11. Recommend Wednesday or Thursday night to prepare and pack the **Smashed Chickpea Dill Sandwich** (page 141), **Tajin Baked Red Potatoes** (page 257), and **Pecan Pie Yogurt Bowl** (page 270) for Friday.
12. Prepare the **PB & Raspberry Shake** (page 100) right before eating.

Meal Plan 3

For: 35-year-old man
Weight: 210 pounds
Exercise: 1 hour, 4 to 5 days a week
Calories: 2,550

Protein needs: 1.4g/kg body weight = **133 grams per day**
Diet: Omnivore

	Monday	Tuesday-Thursday	Friday
Breakfast	**Apple-Walnut Cottage Cheese Bowls** *Total Calories: 285* *Carbohydrates: 15g* *Protein: 17g* *Fat: 15g*		**Green Protein Shake** *Total Calories: 401* *Carbohydrates: 41g* *Protein: 18g* *Fat: 19g*
Morning Snack	**Cottage Cheese-Blueberry Muffins** *Total Calories: 222* *Carbohydrates: 29g* *Protein: 12g* *Fat: 7g*	**Double Chocolate Banana Dream Shake** *Total Calories: 305* *Carbohydrates: 45g* *Protein: 25g* *Fat: 3g*	**Meatballs with Tart Cherry Sauce** **Tajin Baked Red Potatoes** *Total Calories: 424* *Carbohydrates: 39g* *Protein: 21g* *Fat: 21g*
Lunch	**Peanut-Flavored Slaw with Sautéed Chicken** *Total Calories: 494* *Carbohydrates: 27g* *Protein: 39g* *Fat: 28g*	**Peanut-Flavored Slaw with Sautéed Chicken** **1 medium dinner roll** **1½ cups sliced strawberries** *Total Calories: 670* *Carbohydrates: 61g* *Protein:449g* *Fat: 31g*	**Rotisserie Chicken Wrap with Homemade Ranch Dressing** **1½ cups sliced strawberries** *Total Calories: 519* *Carbohydrates: 53g* *Protein: 33g* *Fat: 23g*
Afternoon Snack	**PB & Raspberry Shake** *Total Calories: 278* *Carbohydrates: 37g* *Protein: 26g* *Fat: 2g*	**Cottage Cheese-Blueberry Muffins** **2 clementines** *Total Calories: 292* *Carbohydrates: 47g* *Protein: 13g* *Fat: 7g*	**Cottage Cheese-Blueberry Muffins** **2 cups seedless grapes** *Total Calories: 346* *Carbohydrates: 60g* *Protein: 13g* *Fat: 7g*

Dinner	**Herb-Marinated Beef Shish Kebabs** **Couscous with Chickpeas, Peas, and Carrots** **1 medium pear** *Total Calories: 806* *Carbohydrates: 66g* *Protein: 38g* *Fat: 44g*		**Chicken Piccata over Angel Hair** **1 cup steamed broccoli** **Chocolate Cottage Cheese Bark with Nuts** *Total Calories: 804* *Carbohydrates: 73g* *Protein: 50g* *Fat: 33g*
Nutrition Information	*Total Calories: 2,673* *Carbohydrates: 183g* *Protein: 132g* *Fat: 96g* *Carbohydrates: 48%* *Protein: 20%* *Fat: 32%*	*Total Calories: 2,462* *Carbohydrates: 247g* *Protein: 134g* *Fat: 102g* *Carbohydrates: 40%* *Protein: 23%* *Fat: 37%*	*Total Calories: 2552* *Carbohydrates: 267g* *Protein: 135g* *Fat: 104g* *Carbohydrates: 42%* *Protein: 21.5%* *Fat: 36%*

MEAL PLAN 3: RECIPES

- Apple-Walnut Cottage Cheese Bowls (page 119)
- Double Chocolate Banana Dream Shake (page 98)
- Green Protein Shake (page 103)
- Chicken Piccata over Angel Hair (page 208)
- Chocolate Cottage Cheese Bark with Nuts (page 279)
- Cottage Cheese-Blueberry Muffins (page 272)
- Couscous with Chickpeas, Peas, and Carrots (page 255)
- Herb-Marinated Beef Shish Kebabs (page 228)
- Meatballs with Tart Cherry Sauce (page 265)
- PB & Raspberry Shake (page 100)
- Peanut-Flavored Slaw with Sautéed Chicken (page 134)
- Rotisserie Chicken Wrap with Homemade Ranch Dressing (page 147)
- Tajin Baked Red Potatoes (page 257)

MEAL PLAN 3: SHOPPING LIST

PANTRY

- Almond butter
- Almonds, dry-roasted unsalted
- Angel hair (1 × 1-pound box)
- Baking powder
- Baking soda
- Basil, dried
- Black pepper, ground
- Breadcrumbs, unseasoned
- Broth, low-sodium chicken
- Broth, low-sodium vegetable
- Capers
- Cayenne pepper
- Chickpeas, low-sodium (1 × 15.5-ounce can)
- Chocolate, 60 percent dark (1 × 8-ounce bar)
- Cinnamon, ground
- Cocoa, unsweetened
- Cooking spray, nonstick
- Couscous
- Cumin, ground
- Fish sauce
- Flaxseed meal
- Flour, all-purpose
- Garlic powder
- Ginger, ground
- Honey
- Hot sauce or sriracha
- Italian seasoning
- Juice, apple, 100 percent
- Maple syrup, pure
- Marjoram, dried
- Mayonnaise, light
- Mustard, Dijon
- Mustard powder
- Oats, rolled
- Oil, canola
- Oil, extra-virgin olive
- Oil, olive
- Onion powder
- Oregano, dried
- Paprika, smoked
- Peanut butter powder
- Peanut butter, smooth
- Peanuts, dry-roasted, unsalted
- Pine nuts
- Pistachios, dry-roasted unsalted
- Roll, small dinner (3)
- Rosemary, dried
- Sage, ground
- Salt, kosher
- Salt, sea
- Salt, table
- Skewers (16)
- Soy sauce, reduced sodium
- Sugar, dark brown
- Sugar, granulated
- Sunflower seeds, dry roasted, unsalted
- Tajin seasoning
- Thyme, dried
- Tomato paste (1 × 6-ounce can)
- Vinegar, balsamic
- Vinegar, red wine
- Whey protein isolate, unflavored (25g protein per 1 scoop)
- Wine, white cooking or dry white
- Worcestershire sauce

FRUIT, VEGETABLES, HERBS & SPICES

- Apple, Honeycrisp, Cosmic Crisp, Granny Smith, or Fuji (1)
- Banana, medium (6)
- Bean sprouts
- Broccoli (1 cup)
- Cabbage, red
- Carrots
- Chives
- Cilantro
- Garlic, bulb (2)
- Lemon (3)
- Lime (2)
- Onion, green (1 bunch)
- Onion, yellow, small (2)

- Onion, yellow, medium (1)
- Parsley, flat-leaf
- Pepper, jalapeño (1)
- Pepper, red bell
- Potatoes, red (1½ pounds, about 4 medium)
- Shallot (1)
- Spinach, baby
- Strawberries (6 cups)
- Tomato, cherry

PROTEIN

- Beef, ground, at least 90 percent lean (1 pound)
- Beef sirloin, like top sirloin (1½ pounds)
- Chicken, rotisserie
- Chicken, skinless, boneless breast (1 pound)
- Chicken, skinless, boneless breast, thin sliced (1⅓ pounds)
- Eggs, large (3)

DAIRY

- Butter, unsalted
- Buttermilk, low-fat
- Cottage cheese, 2 percent (3¾ cups)
- Kefir, low-fat vanilla
- Milk, ultra-filtered (1 × 52-ounce bottle)
- Yogurt, Greek, nonfat vanilla (½ cup)
- Yogurt, Greek, reduced-fat plain (single-serve cup)

FROZEN

- Blueberries
- Cherries, pitted sweet dark or tart cherries
- Peas and carrots
- Pineapple chunks
- Raspberries

MEAL PLAN 3: STEP-BY-STEP PREP

1. Prepare the **Chicken Piccata over Angel Hair** and pack to freeze (page 208).
2. Prepare the **Cottage Cheese-Blueberry Muffins,** steps 1 to 7 (page 272).
3. While the muffins are baking, prepare the **Apple-Walnut Cottage Cheese Bowls** (page 119).
4. Package the **Cottage Cheese-Blueberry Muffins,** step 8 (page 272).
5. Prepare the **Herb-Marinated Beef Shish Kebabs,** step 1 (page 228).
6. While the beef is marinating, prepare the **Couscous with Chickpeas, Peas, and Carrots** (page 255).

7. Cook the **Herb-Marinated Beef Shish Kebabs,** steps 2 to 7 (page 228).
8. Prepare the **Meatballs with Tart Cherry Sauce** and pack to freeze (page 265).
9. Prepare the **Peanut-Flavored Slaw with Sautéed Chicken** (page 134) and steam the broccoli.
10. Prepare the **Chocolate Cottage Cheese Bark with Nuts** (page 279).
11. On Wednesday or Thursday, prepare the **Tajin Baked Red Potatoes,** steps 1 to 3 (page 257) and **Rotisserie Chicken Wrap with Homemade Ranch Dressing** (page 147) for Friday.
12. Prepare the **Double Chocolate Banana Dream Shake** (page 98) and **Green Protein Shake** (page 103) right before eating.

Meal Plan 4

For: 35-year-old woman
Weight: 150 pounds
Exercise: Most days of the week for 1 hour

Calories: 2,000
Protein needs: 1.6g/kg body weight = **108 grams per day**
Diet: Omnivore

	Monday–Thursday	Friday
Breakfast	Black Beans and Eggs Breakfast Bowl *Total Calories: 398* *Carbohydrates: 42g* *Protein: 20g* *Fat: 21g*	Green Protein Shake *Total Calories: 401* *Carbohydrates: 41g* *Protein: 26g* *Fat: 18g*
Morning Snack	Cottage Cheese-Blueberry Muffins ¼ cup dried apricot halves *Total Calories: 300* *Carbohydrates: 49g* *Protein: 13g* *Fat: 7g*	Cottage Cheese-Blueberry Muffins *Total Calories: 222* *Carbohydrates: 29g* *Protein: 12g* *Fat: 7g*

	Monday - Thursday	Friday
Lunch	**Rotisserie Chicken Wrap with Homemade Ranch Dressing** **Tajin Baked Red Potatoes** *Total Calories: 618* *Carbohydrates: 60g* *Protein: 34g* *Fat: 29g*	**Chopped Salad with Chickpeas and Tuna** **Whole wheat pita** **1 cup diced pineapple** *Total Calories: 529* *Carbohydrates: 59g* *Protein: 32g* *Fat: 17g*
Afternoon Snack	**Spicy Black Bean Dip** *Total Calories: 127* *Carbohydrates: 22g* *Protein: 8g* *Fat: 1g*	**Chocolate Cottage Cheese Bark with Nuts** *Total Calories: 230* *Carbohydrates: 18g* *Protein: 6g* *Fat: 15g*
Dinner	**Chicken Stir-Fry with Broccoli, Snow Peas, and Mushrooms** **1 orange** *Total Calories: 572* *Carbohydrates: 62g* *Protein: 34g* *Fat: 17g*	**Tomato-Basil Chicken Thighs and Rice** **Lemon-Garlic Spinach** *Total Calories: 481* *Carbohydrates: 49g* *Protein: 39g* *Fat: 3g*
Nutrition Information	*Total Calories: 2,063* *Carbohydrates: 237g* *Protein: 110g* *Fat: 75g* *Carbohydrates: 46%* *Protein: 21%* *Fat: 33%*	*Total Calories: 1,990* *Carbohydrates: 212g* *Protein: 110g* *Fat: 78g* *Carbohydrates: 43%* *Protein: 22%* *Fat: 35%*

MEAL PLAN 4: RECIPES

- Black Beans and Eggs Breakfast Bowl (page 124)
- Chicken Stir-Fry with Broccoli, Snow Peas, and Mushrooms (page 216)
- Chocolate Cottage Cheese Bark with Nuts (page 279)
- Chopped Salad with Chickpeas and Tuna (page 145)
- Cottage Cheese-Blueberry Muffins (page 272)
- Green Protein Shake (page 103)
- Lemon-Garlic Spinach (page 251)

- Rotisserie Chicken Wrap with Homemade Ranch Dressing (page 147)
- Spicy Black Bean Dip (page 263)
- Tajin Baked Red Potatoes (page 257)
- Tomato-Basil Chicken Thighs and Rice (page 210)

MEAL PLAN 4: SHOPPING LIST

PANTRY

- Almond butter
- Almonds, dry-roasted unsalted
- Apple, juice, 100 percent
- Baking powder
- Baking soda
- Balsamic vinegar
- Beans, low-sodium black (3 × 15.5-ounce cans)
- Black pepper, ground
- Broth, low-sodium chicken
- Broth, low-sodium vegetable
- Cayenne pepper
- Chickpeas, low-sodium (1 × 15.5-ounce can)
- Chili powder
- Chocolate, 60 percent dark chocolate (1 × 8-ounce bar)
- Cooking spray, nonstick
- Coriander seed, ground
- Cornstarch
- Cumin, ground
- Flaxseed meal
- Flour, all-purpose
- Mayonnaise, light
- Nutritional yeast
- Oats, rolled
- Oil, canola
- Oil, extra-virgin olive
- Oil, olive
- Oregano, dried
- Paprika, smoked
- Parsley, dried
- Peppers, roasted red
- Pistachios, dry-roasted unsalted
- Pita, whole wheat (1)
- Red pepper flakes
- Rice, basmati white
- Rice, Jasmine
- Salt, kosher
- Salt, sea
- Salt, table
- Sugar, granulated
- Tajin seasoning
- Thyme, dried
- Tomatoes, fire-roasted diced (1 × 14.5-ounce can)
- Tortillas, whole wheat (4)
- Tuna, albacore tuna packed in water (2 × 5-ounce cans)
- Whey protein isolate (25g protein per 1 scoop)
- Wine, cooking or dry white

FRUIT, VEGETABLES, HERBS & SPICES

- Avocado (2)
- Basil leaves
- Broccoli florets (2 cups)
- Carrots, baby
- Celery
- Chives
- Cilantro
- Cucumber, hothouse (1)
- Garlic, bulb (2)
- Lemon (3)
- Lime (2)
- Mushrooms, white button (1 × 8 ounce package)
- Onion, red, small (1)
- Onion, yellow, medium (2)

- Onion, yellow, small (1)
- Oranges (4)
- Parsley, flat-leaf
- Pepper, green bell (1)
- Pepper, jalapeño (3)
- Pepper, red bell (1)
- Pepper, yellow or orange bell (1)
- Potatoes, red, 1½ pounds (4 medium)
- Pineapple (1)
- Scallions (1 bunch)
- Snow peas (1 cup)
- Spinach, baby (1 pound + 1 cup)
- Tomato, cherry
- Tomato, plum (2)

PROTEIN

- Chicken, breast, skinless, boneless (1 pound)
- Chicken, rotisserie
- Chicken, thighs, boneless, skinless (1½ pounds)
- Eggs, large (6)

DAIRY

- Butter, unsalted
- Buttermilk, low fat
- Cheese, Cotija (3 ounces)
- Cheese, feta, crumbled
- Cheese, reduced fat pepper jack or cheddar
- Cottage cheese, reduced-fat 2 percent (1¾ cup)
- Milk, ultra-filtered (1 × 52-ounce bottle)
- Yogurt, Greek, reduced-fat (2 percent), plain

FROZEN

- Blueberries
- Edamame, unshelled
- Pineapple chunks

MEAL PLAN 4: STEP-BY-STEP PREP

1. Prepare the **Tomato-Basil Chicken Thighs and Rice,** steps 1 to 4 (page 210).
2. Pack the **Tomato-Basil Chicken Thighs and Rice,** steps 5 to 7, and freeze (page 210).
3. Prepare the **Black Bean and Eggs Breakfast Bowls** (page 124).
4. Prepare the **Chicken Stir-Fry with Broccoli, Snow Peas, and Mushrooms** (page 216).
5. Prepare the **Chocolate Cottage Cheese Bark with Nuts** (page 279).
6. Prepare the **Cottage Cheese-Blueberry Muffins,** steps 1 to 7 (page 272).
7. While the muffins are baking, prepare the **Lemon-Garlic Spinach** (page 251) and freeze.
8. Pack the **Cottage Cheese-Blueberry Muffins,** step 8 (page 272).

9. Prepare the **Tajin Baked Red Potatoes,** steps 1 to 3 (page 257).
10. While the potatoes are baking, prepare the **Spicy Black Bean Dip** (page 263) and hard boil the eggs.
11. Pack the **Tajin Baked Red Potatoes,** step 5 (page 257).
12. Prepare the **Rotisserie Chicken Wrap with Homemade Ranch Dressing** (page 147).
13. On Wednesday or Thursday, prepare and pack the **Chopped Salad with Chickpeas and Tuna** (page 145), cook the edamame, and dice the pineapple.
14. Prepare the **Green Protein Shake** (page 103) right before eating.

Make-Ahead Strategies for a Busy Weekend

The four meal plans in this chapter were created to meal prep for a busy work-week. But what if you have a busy weekend ahead? Don't stress! I've got you covered. Below are five strategies to plan ahead for that busy weekend.

HAVE A MINI PREP DAY DURING THE WEEK.

Use one or a couple of hours on Wednesday or Thursday to prepare some Friday meals that can last through the weekend. Since leftover food only lasts four days max, prep one or two dishes during a weeknight that can last you through the busy weekend.

COOK AND FREEZE.

If you make a double batch of a dish, a busy weekend is the perfect time to transfer a container to the refrigerator to defrost. That way you will have one or several meals ready to heat and eat over the weekend.

PREPARE INGREDIENTS BEFORE THE WEEKEND.

If you need to decrease your prep time over the weekend, take a little time Thursday night or Friday morning to chop, mince, slice, or dice any ingredients. This can help shave off 10 to 30 minutes of your prep time.

PLAN YOUR MEAL WHEN DINING OUT.

If you're heading out to a party or restaurant over the weekend, check the restaurant's menu online so you can plan your meal and your overall day ahead.

If you're hitting a friend's party, ask what will be served so you know where you will get your protein from.

PREPARE SNACK BOXES.

In chapter 5, there are two Grab-and-Go Protein Boxes (page 108). Prepare these ahead of time so when you don't have time to prepare something, you'll be covered.

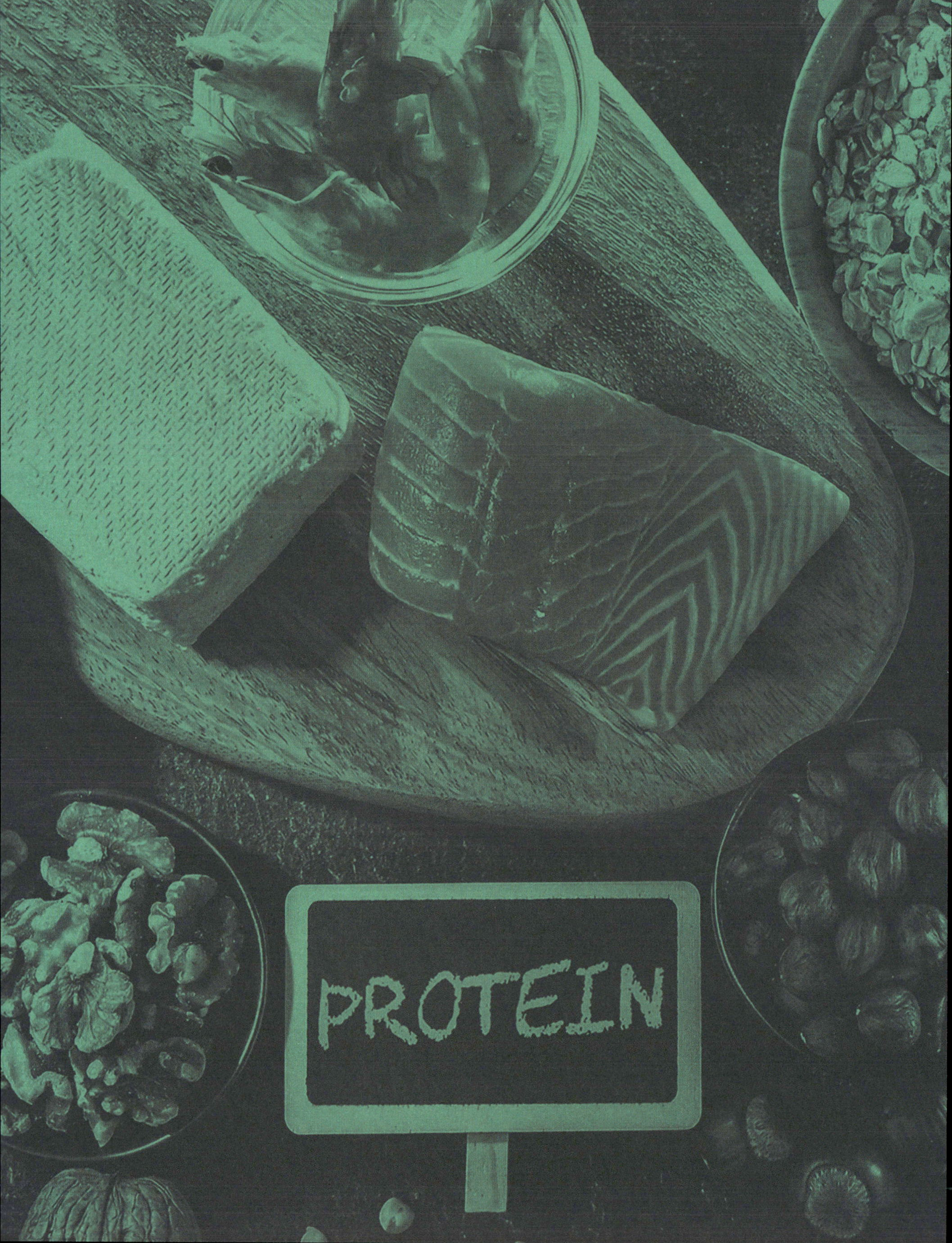
PROTEIN

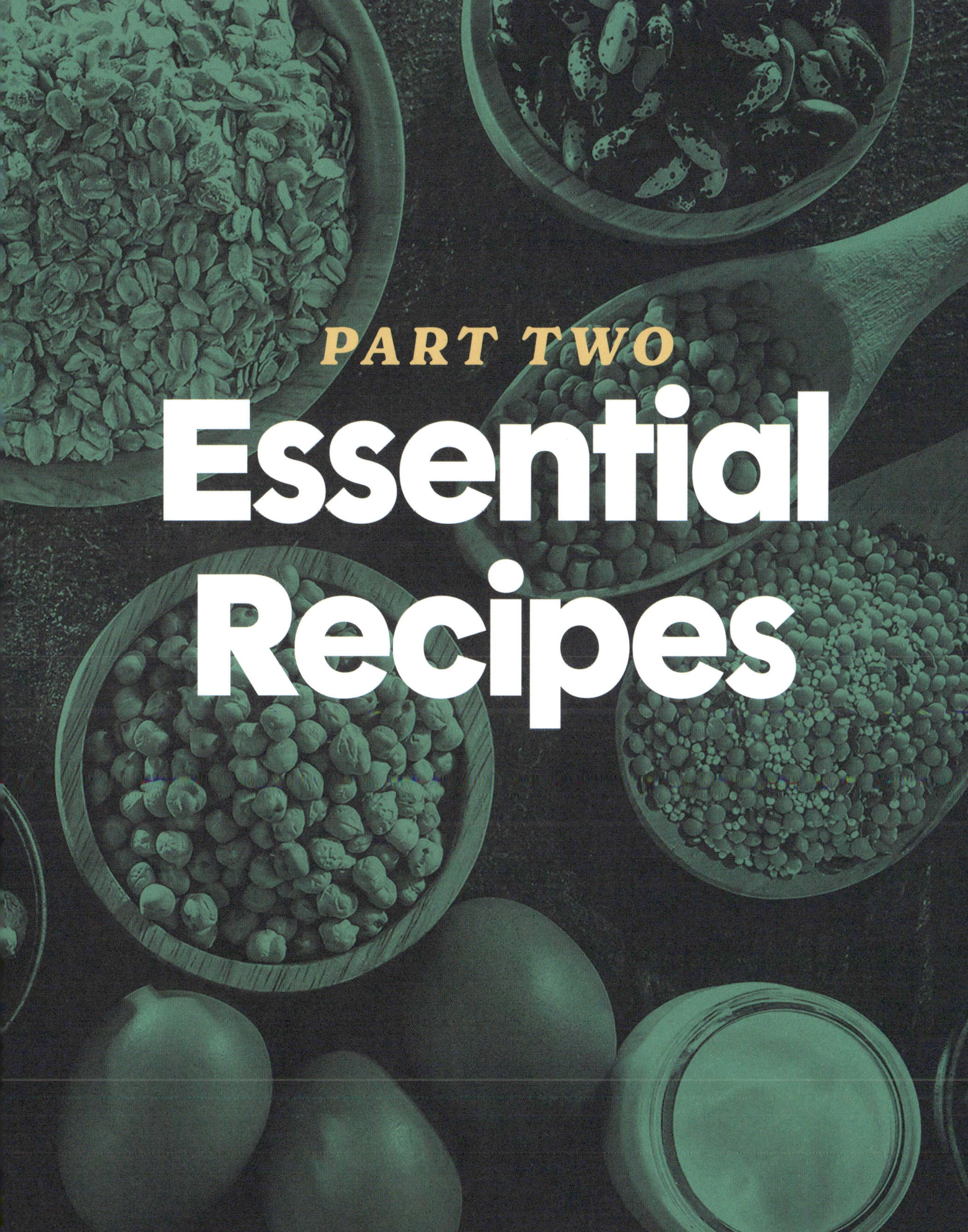

PART TWO

Essential Recipes

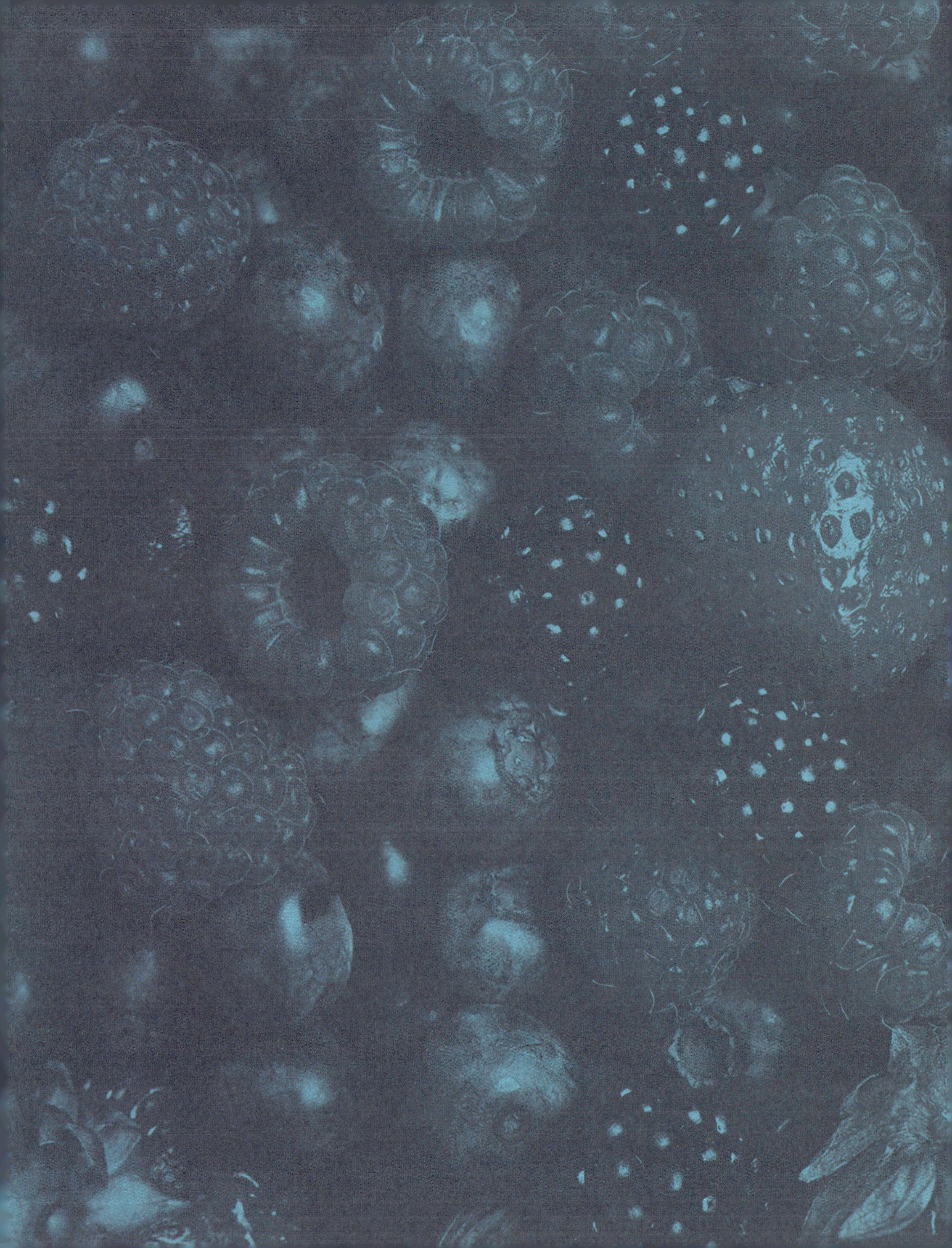

CHAPTER 4

Smoothies and Shakes

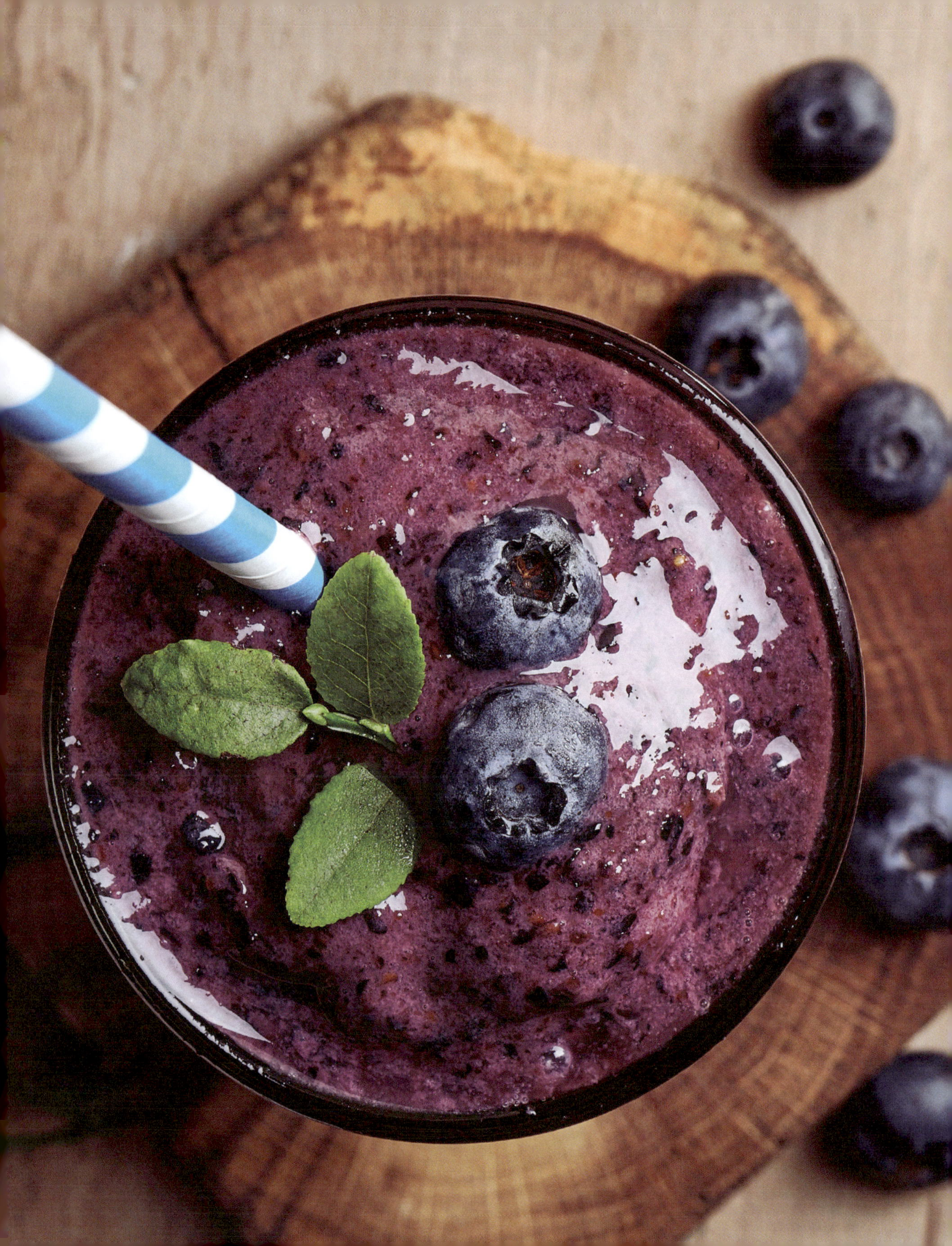

Wild Blueberry Power Smoothie

This satiating protein blend is made with wild blueberries, which contain two times more antioxidants compared to traditional blueberries. These mighty berries are packed with anthocyanins, a natural plant compound that gives them their deep purplish hue and have been shown to help fight inflammation.

PREP TIME 5 min // **COOK TIME** 0 min // **TOTAL TIME** 5 min // **SERVINGS** 1 // **SERVING SIZE** 1¾ cups

One Pot/Pan, 30 Minutes or Less | **Vegetarian, Gluten-Free**

- ½ cup frozen wild blueberries
- ½ cup frozen riced cauliflower
- ½ medium banana
- ½ cup 2 percent cottage cheese
- ½ cup ultra-filtered skim milk (13 grams protein per 1 cup serving)
- 1 teaspoon ground hemp seeds
- ⅛ teaspoon ground cinnamon

1. Place the ingredients in a blender. Cover and blend on high speed until smooth, about 1 minute.
2. *To serve:* Pour into a tall glass and drink immediately.

Nutrition Information (per serving): Calories 275; Total Fat 4g; Saturated Fat 1g; Protein 24g; Total Carbohydrates 35g; Fiber 9g; Total Sugars 15g (Includes Added Sugars 0g); Sodium 118mg

Toby's Tip: Wild blueberries are smaller and sweeter than traditional blueberries and are most commonly found in the frozen fruit section. Swap in traditional blueberries, if needed.

Strawberry Oat Smoothie

This blush-colored smoothie uses silken tofu, which carries any flavor you mix with it. The result is a protein-filled, subtly flavored strawberry smoothie that is perfect for when you are on the go.

PREP TIME 15 min // **COOK TIME** 0 min // **TOTAL TIME** 15 min // **SERVINGS** 1 // **SERVING SIZE** 1¾ cups

One Pot/Pan, 30 Minutes or Less | Vegan, Vegetarian, Gluten-Free, Dairy-Free

- 2 tablespoons certified gluten-free rolled oats
- 1 cup unsweetened soy milk
- 1 cup frozen strawberries
- 3 ounces silken tofu (about ⅓ cup)
- 1 tablespoon ground hemp seeds
- 2 teaspoons agave syrup
- ½ teaspoon pure vanilla extract

1. Place the rolled oats and soy milk into the blender jar and stir with a spoon to combine. Allow the oats to hydrate for at least 10 minutes or up to 30 minutes.
2. Add the strawberries, tofu, hemp seeds, agave, and vanilla to the blender. Cover and blend on high speed until smooth, about 1 minute.
3. *To serve:* Pour into a tall glass and drink immediately.

Nutrition Information (per serving): Calories 329; Total Fat 7g; Saturated Fat 1g; Protein 15g; Total Carbohydrates 53g; Fiber 8g; Total Sugars 25g (Includes Added Sugars 9g); Sodium 95mg

Toby's Tip: Look for "gluten-free" on the oats label. Although oats are naturally gluten-free, they can be processed in a facility with gluten-filled foods.

Cherry Kale Smoothie

The sweet and tart flavor of cherries balance the earthiness of kale, providing a satisfying beverage. It's also another way to get more veggies—and a bit more protein—any time of day.

PREP TIME 5 min // **COOK TIME** 0 min // **TOTAL TIME** 5 min // **SERVINGS** 1 // **SERVING SIZE** 1¾ cups

One Pot/Pan, 30 Minutes or Less | Vegetarian, Gluten-Free

- 1 cup frozen pitted sweet cherries
- 2 cups loosely packed kale leaves, chopped
- ½ cup ultra-filtered skim milk (13 grams protein per serving)
- 1 (19.5-gram) scoop sweetened vanilla whey protein powder (15 grams protein per scoop)

1. Place the ingredients in a blender. Cover and blend on high speed until smooth, about 1 minute.
2. *To serve:* Pour into a tall glass and drink immediately.

Nutrition Information (per serving): Calories 261; Total Fat 2g; Saturated Fat 1g; Protein 26g; Total Carbohydrates 38g; Fiber 5g; Total Sugars 22g (Includes Added Sugars 0g); Sodium 239mg

Toby's Tip: For this smoothie, I use a sweetened protein powder with no added sugar. If you choose to use an unsweetened whey protein powder you may need to add a touch of sweetness from honey, agave syrup, maple syrup, or a low- or no-calorie sweetener like Stevia or monk fruit.

Double Chocolate Banana Dream Shake

This smoothie is packed with nutritional benefits from its four key ingredients. Banana provides potassium, vitamin B6, fiber, and vitamin C, while whey protein powder delivers a dose of protein. Kefir, a fermented dairy beverage, supports gut health with live, active microorganisms plus protein, calcium, and B vitamins, and cocoa offers powerful antioxidant flavonoids.

PREP TIME 5 min // **COOK TIME** 0 min // **TOTAL TIME** 5 min // **SERVINGS** 1 // **SERVING SIZE** 1¾ cups

One Pot/Pan, 30 Minutes or Less | **Vegetarian, Gluten-Free**

1 medium banana

¾ cup unsweetened low-fat vanilla kefir

1 (20.5-gram) scoop sweetened chocolate whey protein powder (15 grams protein per scoop)

1 tablespoon unsweetened cocoa

1. Place the ingredients in a blender. Cover and blend on high speed until smooth, about 1 minute.
2. *To serve:* Pour into a tall glass and drink immediately.

Nutrition Information (per serving): Calories 305; Total Fat 3g; Saturated Fat 2g; Protein 25g; Total Carbohydrates 45g; Fiber 5g; Total Sugars 28g (Includes Added Sugars 8g); Sodium 180mg

Toby's Tip: Kefir is a slightly tangy fermented dairy beverage that tastes great in all types of smoothies. Feel free to swap it for Greek yogurt or use it as a base when making other smoothies.

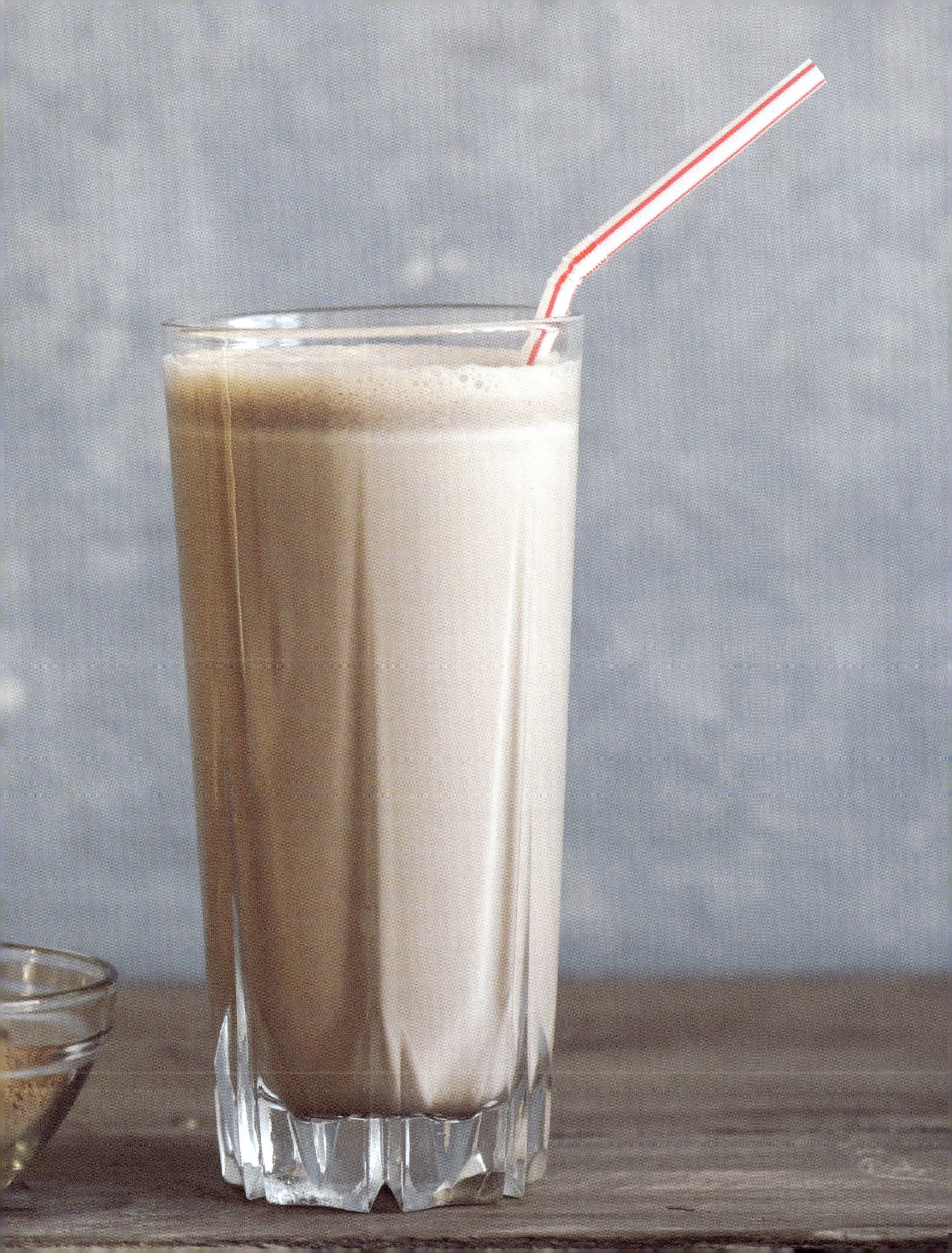

PB & Raspberry Shake

By using ultra-filtered milk, you increase the protein from 8 grams per 1 cup serving in traditional milk to 13 grams. It's a simple way to up your protein—plus, most ultra-filtered milk is lactose-free (check the label).

PREP TIME 5 min // **COOK TIME** 0 min // **TOTAL TIME** 5 min // **SERVINGS** 1 // **SERVING SIZE** 1¾ cups

One Pot/Pan, 30 Minutes or Less | Vegetarian, Gluten-Free

1 cup frozen raspberries

2 tablespoons peanut butter powder (6 grams protein per serving)

¾ cup ultra-filtered skim milk (13 grams protein per 1 cup serving)

½ cup vanilla nonfat Greek yogurt

¼ teaspoon ground cinnamon

1. Place the ingredients in a blender. Cover and blend on high speed until smooth, about 1 minute.
2. *To serve:* Pour into a tall glass and drink immediately.

Nutrition Information (per serving): Calories 278; Total Fat 2g; Saturated Fat 0g; Protein 26g; Total Carbohydrates 37g; Fiber 6g; Total Sugars 24g (Includes Added Sugars 7g); Sodium 220mg

Toby's Tip: Peanut butter powder is made by roasting peanuts, pressing out much of the oil, and grinding the remaining part into a fine powder filled with natural protein from the peanuts. It is not the same as a peanut butter–flavored protein powder. You can typically find it in the peanut butter and jelly aisle or on online markets like Amazon.

Matcha Shake

Matcha is a finely ground powder of processed green tea leaves, known for its vibrant green color, rich umami flavor, and high concentration of antioxidants. It also provides L-theanine, a non-protein amino acid that has been linked to helping reduce stress and anxiety without causing drowsiness.

PREP TIME 5 min // **COOK TIME** 0 min // **TOTAL TIME** 5 min // **SERVINGS** 1 // **SERVING SIZE** 1½ cups

One Pot/Pan, 30 Minutes or Less | Vegan, Vegetarian, Gluten-Free, Dairy-Free

- 1 cup unflavored soy milk
- 1 cup loosely packed kale leaves, chopped
- 1 kiwifruit, peeled
- ½ cup mango, fresh or frozen
- 1 tablespoon almond butter
- 1 tablespoon ground chia seeds
- 2 teaspoons matcha powder
- 2 teaspoons unsweetened shredded coconut
- ½ teaspoon pure vanilla extract

1. Place the ingredients in a blender. Cover and blend on high speed until smooth, about 1 minute.
2. *To serve:* Pour into a tall glass and drink immediately.

Nutrition Information (per serving): Calories 409; Total Fat 18g; Saturated Fat 3g; Protein 19g; Total Carbohydrates 18g; Fiber 15g; Total Sugars 25g (Includes Added Sugars 0g), Sodium 190mg

Toby's Tip: Matcha powder can be pricey, but a little goes a long way. You can swap it for less expensive options like green tea powder, spirulina powder, moringa powder, or coffee powder (which will add caffeine).

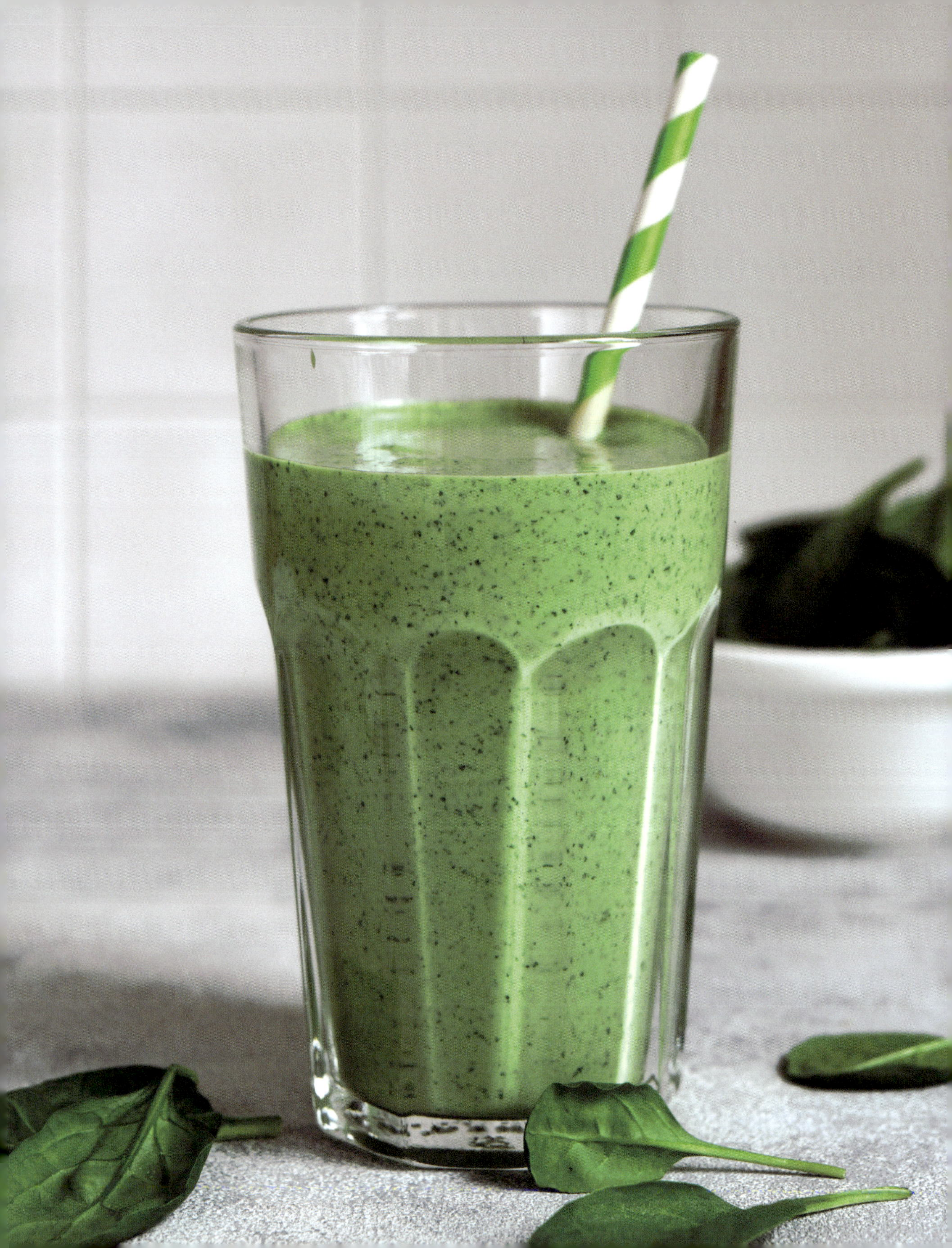

Green Protein Shake

Skip the protein powder. By combining ultra-filtered milk, almond butter, and flaxseed meal, this smoothie uses whole foods to deliver an impressive 18 grams of protein per serving, helping you stay full and satisfied.

PREP TIME 5 min // **COOK TIME** 0 min // **TOTAL TIME** 5 min // **SERVINGS** 1 // **SERVING SIZE** 1½ cups

One Pot/Pan, 30 Minutes or Less | **Vegetarian, Gluten-Free**

- 1 cup loosely packed baby spinach
- ¾ cup fresh or frozen pineapple chunks
- ½ cup ultra-filtered skim milk (13 grams protein per 1 cup serving)
- ¼ cup 100-percent apple juice
- 2 tablespoons almond butter
- 1 tablespoon ground flaxseed meal

1. Place all ingredients in a blender. Cover and blend on high speed until smooth, about 1 minute.
2. *To serve:* Pour into a tall glass and drink immediately.

Nutrition Information (per serving): Calories 401; Total Fat 19g; Saturated Fat 1g; Protein 18g; Total Carbohydrates 41g; Fiber 9g; Total Sugars 31g (Includes Added Sugars 0g); Sodium 108mg

Toby's Tip: Swap the spinach for kale; swap the almond butter for any nut butter of your choice.

Peaches and Cream Milkshake

Skyr is a thick, protein-rich Icelandic dairy product that is technically a soft cheese but is eaten like yogurt due to its creamy texture and mild, slightly tangy flavor. It contains beneficial live and active cultures that may function as probiotics to help support good gut health. You can add skyr to your smoothies for a high-protein boost.

PREP TIME 5 min // **COOK TIME** 0 min // **TOTAL TIME** 5 min // **SERVINGS** 1 // **SERVING SIZE** 1¾ cups

One Pot/Pan, 30 Minutes or Less | Vegetarian, Gluten-Free

- 1 cup peach slices, fresh or frozen
- ½ cup ultra-filtered skim milk (13 grams protein per 1 cup serving)
- ½ cup vanilla whole milk skyr or Icelandic yogurt
- 2 Medjool dates, pitted
- 1 tablespoon ground chia seeds

1. Place the ingredients in a blender. Cover and blend on high speed until smooth, about 1 minute.
2. *To serve:* Pour into a tall glass and drink immediately.

Nutrition Information (per serving): Calories 373; Total Fat 6g; Saturated Fat 3g; Protein 20g; Total Carbohydrates 66g; Fiber 7g; Total Sugars 54g (Includes Added Sugars 0g); Sodium 114mg

Toby's Tip: Dates are a great way to add natural sweetness to smoothies. Aim for 1 to 2 dates (maximum) per serving.

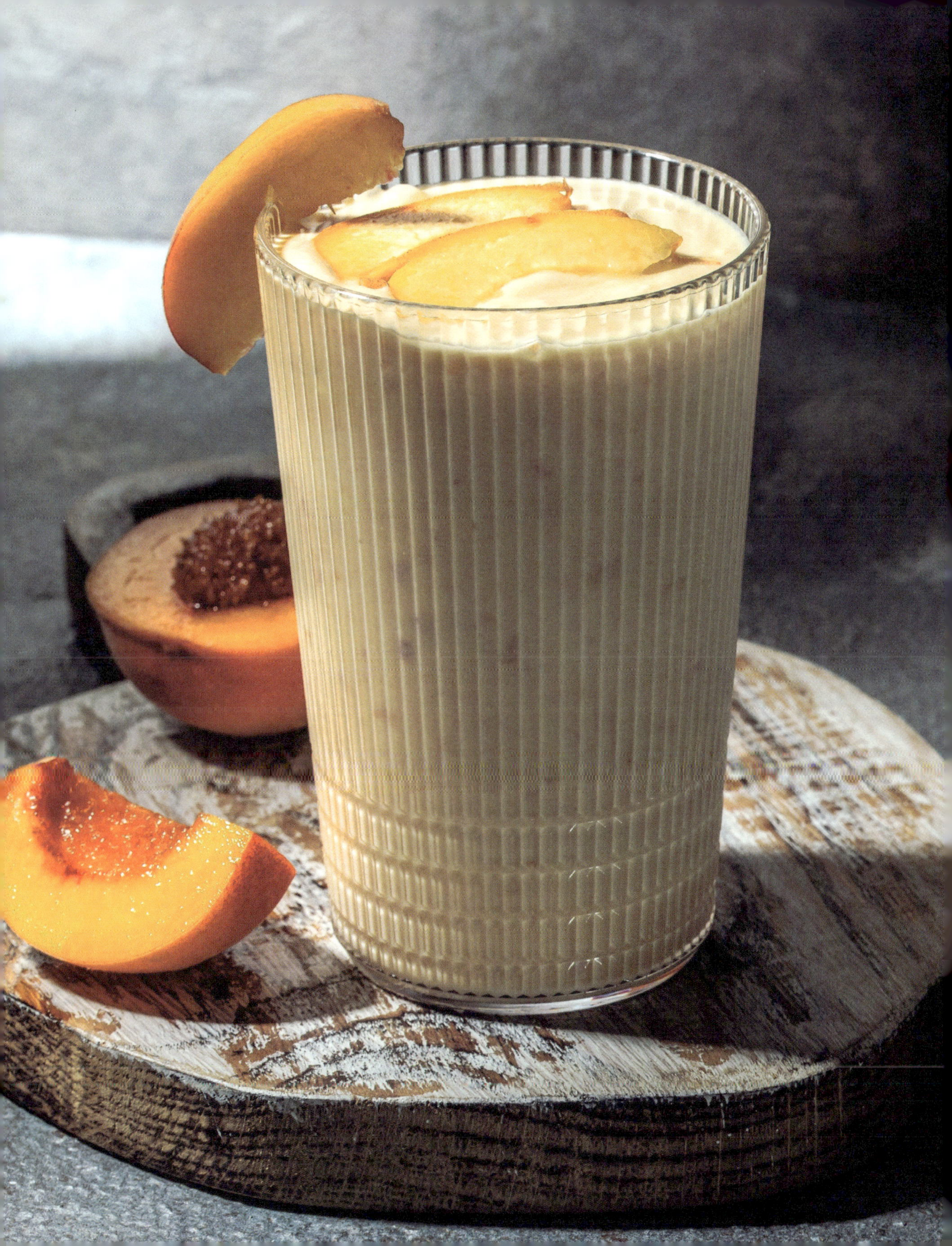

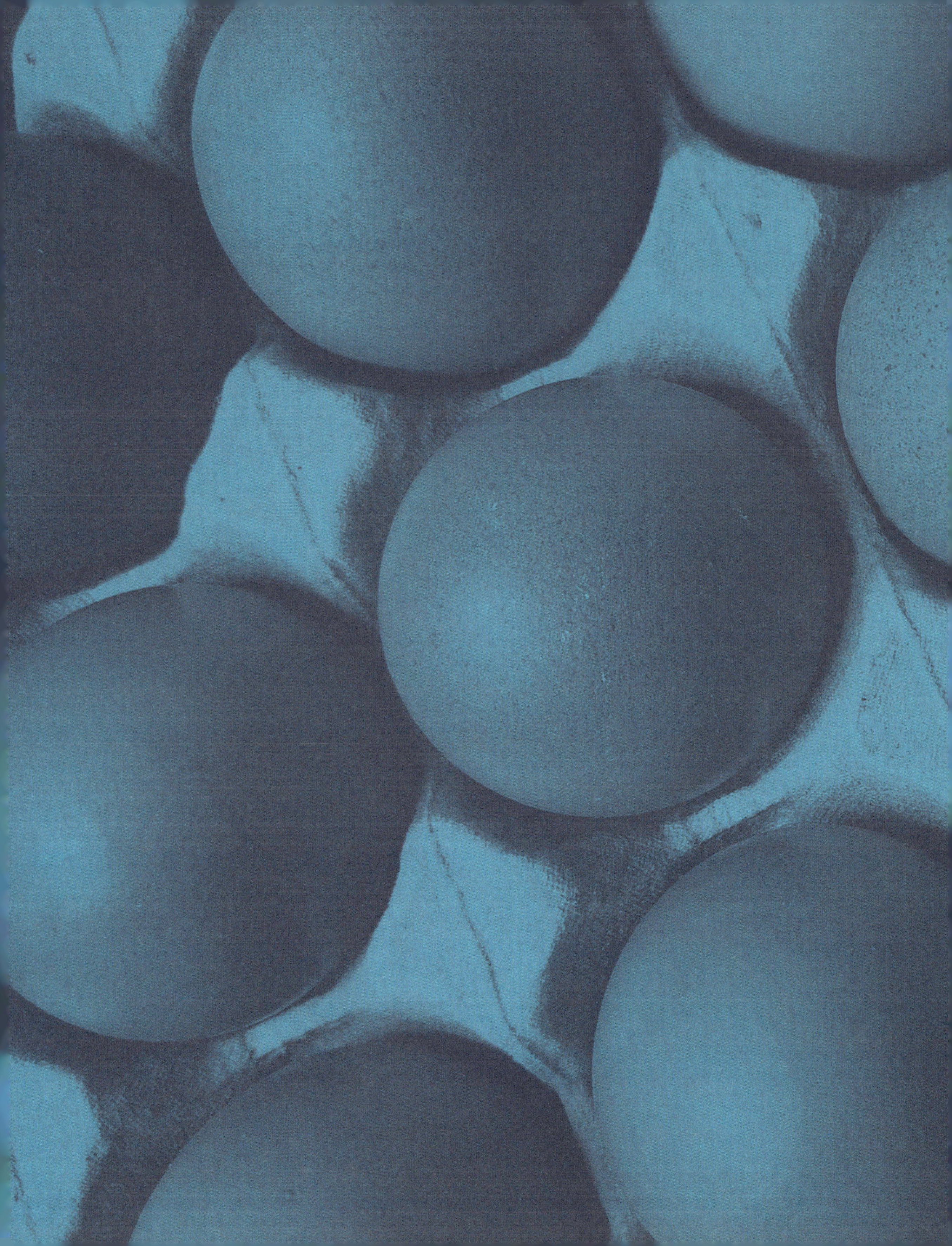

CHAPTER 5

High-Protein Breakfasts

Grab-and-Go Protein Box: Two Ways

Start your week strong by stocking your fridge with these grab-and-go protein boxes. With a healthy, protein-filled meal in your bag, you'll save money and avoid the hassle of unhealthy choices.

Box 1: Egg and Cheese

PREP TIME 25 min // **COOK TIME** 3 min // **TOTAL TIME** 28 min // **SERVINGS** 4 // **SERVING SIZE** 1 box

Meal Prep, 30 Minutes or Less | **Vegetarian**

- 4 large eggs
- 4 ounces reduced-fat cheddar cheese, cubed
- 20 whole-grain crackers (about 120 calories per serving)
- 4 tablespoons peanut butter, smooth or chunky
- 2 cups green or red seedless grapes

1. Place the eggs in a medium saucepan and cover with cold water. Place the saucepan over high heat and bring the water to a boil; cook the eggs for 3 minutes. Remove the saucepan from the heat, cover, and allow to stand for 15 minutes. Drain, and run cold water over the eggs until completely cool, about 10 minutes. Once they have cooled, peel the eggs.
2. *To meal prep:* In each of four compartmental food storage or bento boxes, place 1 hard-boiled egg, 1 ounce cheese, 5 crackers, 1 tablespoon peanut butter, and ½ cup of grapes. Cover boxes and store in the refrigerator for up to four days.

Nutrition Information (per serving): Calories 408; Total Fat 22g; Saturated Fat 8g; Protein 22g; Total Carbohydrates 32g; Fiber 5g; Total Sugars 11g (Includes Added Sugars 0g); Sodium 593mg

Box 2: Cottage Cheese Delight

PREP TIME 15 min // **COOK TIME** 0 min // **TOTAL TIME** 15 min // **SERVINGS** 4 // **SERVING SIZE** 1 box

Meal Prep, 30 Minutes or Less | Vegetarian, Gluten-Free

2 cups 2 percent cottage cheese

2 cups cantaloupe, diced

1 cup unsalted dry-roasted or raw almonds

¼ cup unsalted dry-roasted or raw sunflower seeds

1. *To meal prep:* In each of four compartmental food storage or bento boxes, place ½ cup cottage cheese, ½ cup of cantaloupe, ¼ cup almonds, and 1 tablespoon sunflower seeds. Cover boxes and store in the refrigerator for up to four days.

Nutrition Information (per serving): Calories 377; Total Fat 25g; Saturated Fat 3g; Protein 23g; Total Carbohydrates 20g; Fiber 5g; Total Sugars 12g (Includes Added Sugars 0g); Sodium 387mg

Toby's Tip: Don't forget to stash your to-go boxes in the refrigerator when you get to work or use cold packs to keep them as cold as possible.

Chicken, Pepper, and Mushroom Scramble

Enjoy chicken with your eggs to start your morning on the right foot. You can easily make this scramble with leftover chicken to cut back on prep and cook time—and minimize food waste.

PREP TIME 15 min // **COOK TIME** 15 min // **TOTAL TIME** 30 min // **SERVINGS** 4 // **SERVING SIZE** ~¾ cup

Meal Prep, 30 Minutes or Less | Gluten-Free

- 4 ounces boneless, skinless chicken breast, trimmed and cut into bite-size pieces
- ¼ teaspoon plus ⅛ teaspoon kosher salt, divided
- ¼ teaspoon ground black pepper, divided
- 3 tablespoons olive oil, divided
- 4 large eggs
- 4 large egg whites
- ½ cup ultra-filtered skim milk (13 grams per 1 cup serving)
- ½ teaspoon dried parsley
- ½ red bell pepper, seeds and ribs removed, and finely chopped
- 2 medium button mushrooms, finely chopped
- ½ cup shredded part-skim mozzarella cheese

1. Sprinkle the chicken pieces with ⅛ teaspoon each of the salt and pepper.
2. In a medium skillet, heat 1 tablespoon of the oil over medium heat. Once the oil is shimmering, add the chicken and cook until the internal temperature reaches 165°F, about 5 minutes. Transfer the chicken to a small bowl to slightly cool, about 5 minutes.
3. In a medium bowl, whisk together the eggs, additional egg whites, milk, dried parsley, and the remaining ¼ teaspoon salt and ⅛ teaspoon pepper.
4. Heat the remaining 2 tablespoons of oil in the same skillet over medium heat. Once the oil is shimmering, add the peppers and mushrooms and cook until the vegetables begin to soften, about 5 minutes. Add the cooked chicken and stir to combine. Pour the egg mixture over the vegetables and chicken. Using a spatula, fold and invert the eggs until large, soft curds form, about 4 minutes. Sprinkle with cheese and cook for an additional 30 seconds, until the cheese is slightly melted.
5. *To serve*: Spoon about ¾ cup of the egg scramble onto each of four plates; serve warm.
6. *To meal prep:* Place three-quarters of the egg mixture into each of four resealable containers, cover, and store in the refrigerator for up to 4 days.

7. *To reheat*: Place onto a microwave-safe plate and reheat on high for 45 seconds. Serve warm.

Nutrition Information (per serving): Calories 272; Total Fat 19g; Saturated Fat 5g; Protein 22g; Total Carbohydrates 3g; Fiber 0g; Total Sugars 2g (Includes Added Sugars 0g); Sodium 363mg

Toby's Tip: With 9 grams of protein per ounce of chicken breast, feel free to add a few more ounces to increase the total protein in this meal.

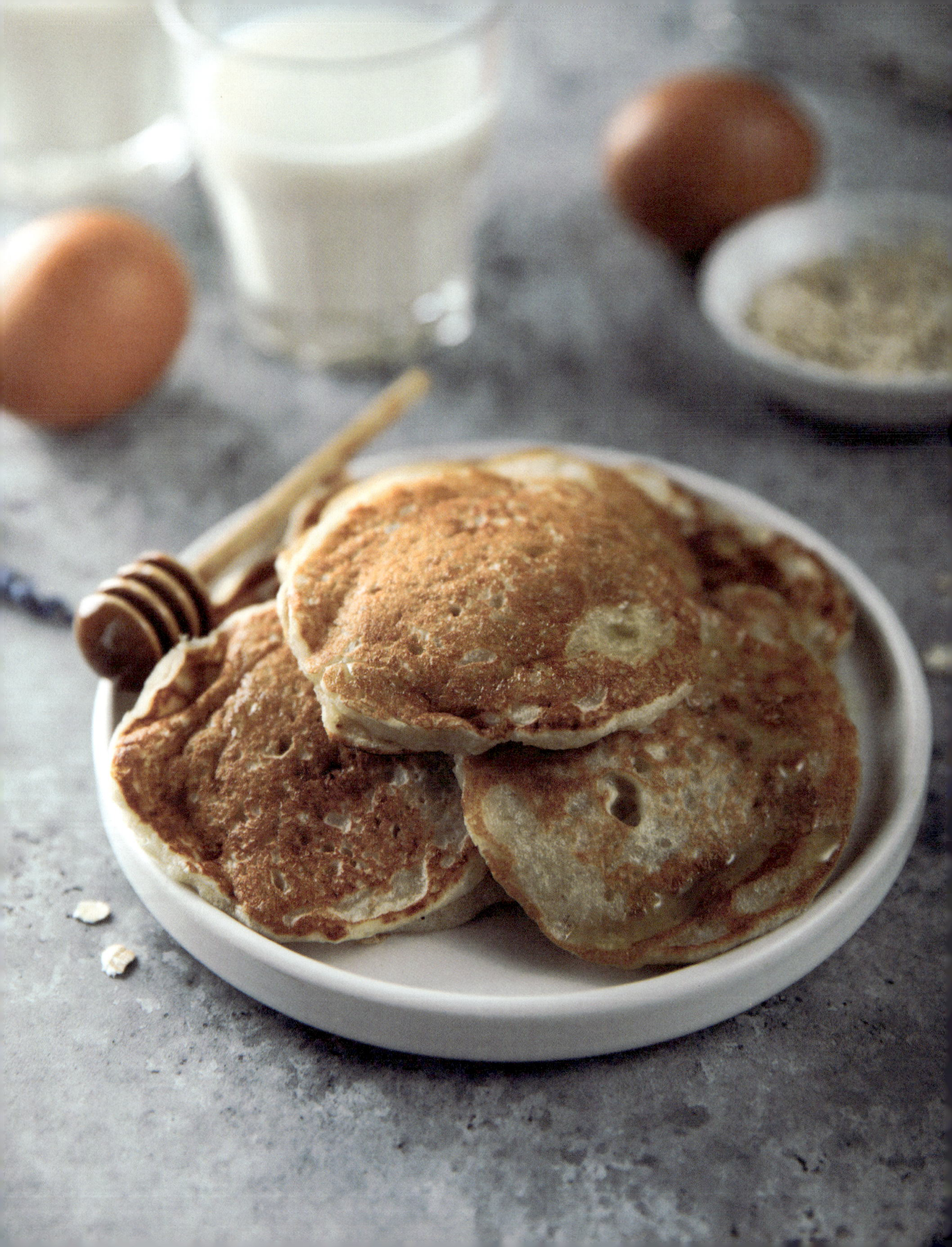

Protein Pancakes *with* Strawberry Yogurt Purée

The secret ingredient in these protein pancakes? Cottage cheese! These babies are so delicious that all leftovers were gobbled up by my daughter's boyfriend, who is always looking for delicious ways to up his protein.

PREP TIME 20 min // **COOK TIME** 10 min // **TOTAL TIME** 30 min // **SERVINGS** 4

SERVING SIZE 2 pancakes with ¼ cup purée

Meal Prep | **Vegetarian, Gluten-Free**

FOR THE STRAWBERRY YOGURT PURÉE

1 cup strawberries, fresh or frozen

¾ cup plain nonfat Greek yogurt

1 tablespoon chia seeds

2 tablespoons lemon juice

1 tablespoon pure maple syrup

FOR THE PANCAKES

1½ cups 2 percent cottage cheese

1 cup gluten-free rolled oats

1 tablespoon flaxseed meal

3 large eggs

2 teaspoons baking powder

1 teaspoon ground cinnamon

1 teaspoon pure vanilla extract

Nonstick cooking spray

1. In a blender, place the strawberries, yogurt, chia seeds, lemon juice, and maple syrup. Cover and blend on high speed for 1 minute. Uncover the blender and, using a rubber spatula, scrape down the sides. Then cover and blend on high speed until smooth, about 30 seconds. Transfer the strawberry mixture to a small bowl. Cover and place in the refrigerator to keep chilled.
2. To a clean blender, add the cottage cheese, rolled oats, flaxseed meal, eggs, baking powder, cinnamon, and vanilla. Cover and blend on high speed until the mixture is smooth, about 1 minute.
3. Coat a large griddle pan with nonstick cooking spray and heat over medium heat. Once the oil is shimmering, pour ⅓ cup of the batter onto the skillet; repeat three more times, spacing pancakes 1 inch apart. Cook until the tops are bubbly and the edges are set, about 3 minutes. Flip the pancakes and cook for another 2 minutes, until golden brown. Transfer to a plate and cover with aluminum foil to keep warm. Repeat with remaining batter.
4. *To serve*: Place 2 pancakes on each of 4 plates. Spoon the purée into each of 4 small bowls and serve on the side for dipping, or spoon on top of the pancakes. Serve immediately.

recipe continues

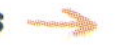

5. *To meal prep:* Place the pancakes into each of 4 resealable containers. Cover and place in the refrigerator. Place ¼ cup purée into each of 4 small separate resealable containers. Store for up to 4 days in the refrigerator.

6. *To reheat:* Place pancakes in a microwave-safe container or on a plate. Heat in the microwave on high for 30 seconds. Top with the purée or serve the purée alongside for dipping.

Nutrition Information (per serving): Calories 285; Total Fat 9g; Saturated Fat 2g; Protein 23g; Total Carbohydrates 29g; Fiber 5g; Total Sugars 10g (Includes Added Sugars 3.5g); Sodium 569mg

Toby's Tip: Swap Greek yogurt with soy yogurt, which has 3 to 9 grams of protein per serving.

Quinoa, Oats, and Seed Porridge

Oats are a star player in the world of healthy breakfasts, packed with fiber that keeps you feeling full and satisfied. To take things up a notch, combine them with protein-filled quinoa, nuts, seeds, and ultra-filtered milk. This warming and nourishing meal is all about providing not only protein but also a variety of good-for-you nutrients.

PREP TIME 15 min // **COOK TIME** 15 min // **TOTAL TIME** 30 min // **SERVINGS** 6 // **SERVING SIZE** 1 bowl

Meal Prep, 30 Minutes or Less | **Vegetarian, Gluten-Free**

- 1 cup gluten-free rolled oats
- ¾ cup dry quinoa
- 2 tablespoons flaxseed meal
- 2 tablespoons pure maple syrup
- 1 teaspoon ground cinnamon
- ¼ teaspoon kosher salt
- 5 ½ cups ultra-filtered skim milk (13 grams protein per 1 cup serving), divided
- ½ cup unsalted dry-roasted pumpkin seeds
- 3 medium bananas, cut into ½-inch moons, divided
- 1 ½ cups fresh blackberries, divided
- ¾ cup unsalted dry-roasted or raw pistachios, roughly chopped, divided

Nutrition Information (per serving): Calories 371; Total Fat 14g; Saturated Fat 2g; Protein 22g; Total Carbohydrates 43g; Fiber 7g; Total Sugars 20g (Includes Added Sugars 4.5g); Sodium 166mg

1. In a medium saucepan, add the oats, quinoa, flaxseed meal, maple syrup, cinnamon, and salt. Pour in 4 cups of the milk and stir to combine.
2. Place the pan over high heat and bring the mixture to a boil. Reduce the heat to medium-low, cover, and cook, stirring occasionally, until the grains are soft and quinoa is fluffy, about 15 minutes. Remove the porridge from the heat and stir in the pumpkin seeds.
3. *To serve:* In each of six bowls, spoon about ½ cup porridge and top with one-sixth of the banana slices, ¼ cup blackberries, and 2 tablespoons pistachios. Top each with ¼ cup of the remaining milk. Serve warm.
4. *To meal prep:* In each of six microwave-safe containers, ladle ½ cup porridge. Place one-sixth of the bananas, ¼ cup blackberries, and 2 tablespoons pistachios in separate smaller containers. Cover the containers and store in the refrigerator for up to 4 days.
5. *To reheat:* Add a splash of milk to a serving of porridge. Heat in the microwave on high for 45 seconds; stir to evenly distribute the heat. Top with the bananas, blackberries, and pistachios and serve.

Toby's Tip: To make the porridge dairy-free but keep much of the protein, substitute the cow's milk with soy milk.

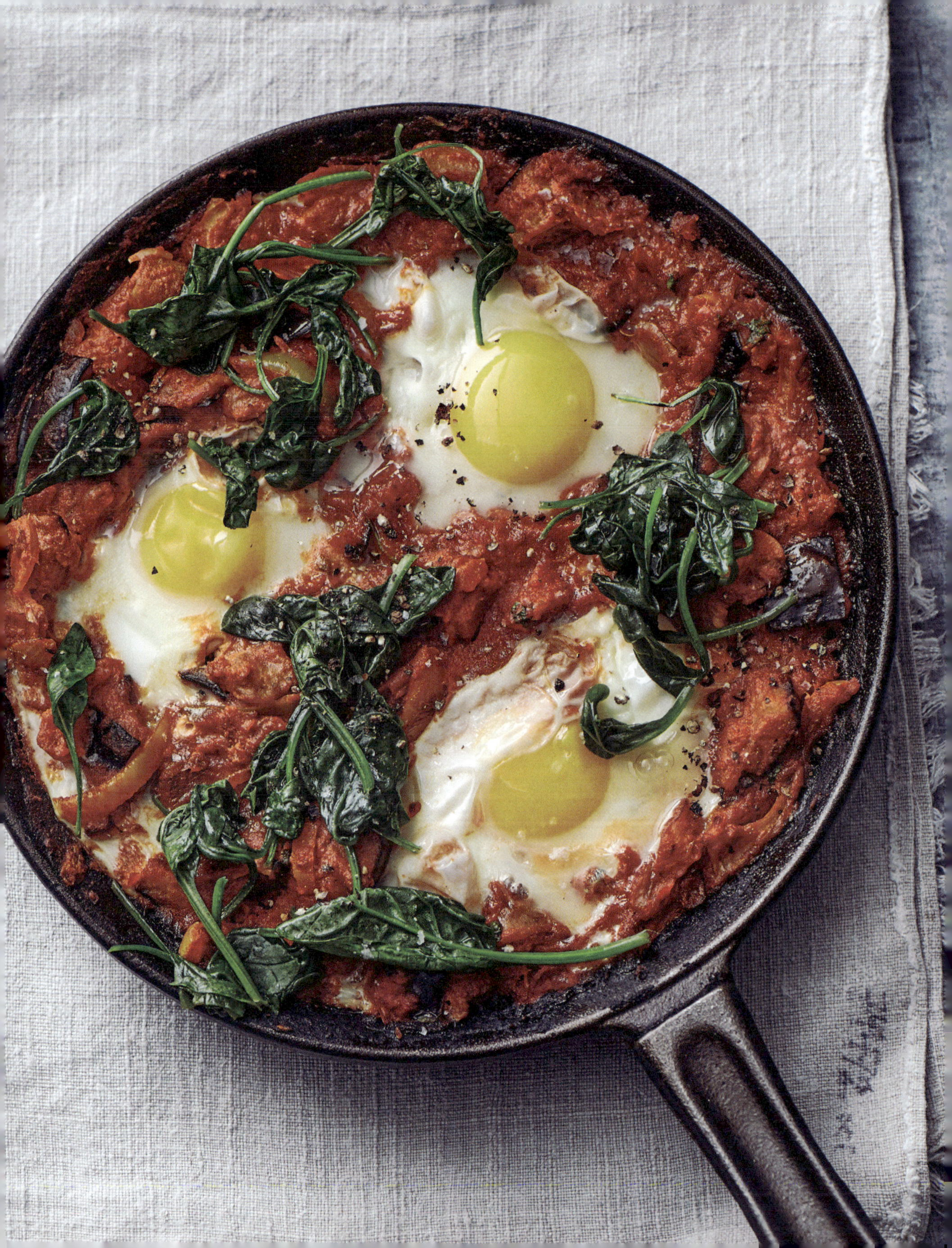

Lentil Shakshuka

This dish, also called "eggs in purgatory," is believed to have originated in Tunisia, though its precise origins are debated. Commonly enjoyed for dinner across the Mediterranean and Middle East, this hearty version simmers lentils directly into the tomato base, creating a thick, protein-rich sauce beneath the eggs.

PREP TIME 15 min // **COOK TIME** 30 min // **TOTAL TIME** 45 min // **SERVINGS** 6

SERVING SIZE: ~1 cup lentil mixture with 1 egg

Meal Prep, Freezer-Friendly | Vegetarian, Gluten-Free

- 1 tablespoon olive oil
- 1 medium yellow onion, cut into ¾-inch-wide slices
- 1 red bell pepper, seeds and core removed, cut into ¾-inch-wide strips
- 2 cloves garlic, minced
- 1 (28-ounce) can crushed tomatoes
- 1 (15-ounce) can brown lentils
- 1 teaspoon ground cumin
- 1 teaspoon sweet paprika
- ⅛ teaspoon cayenne pepper
- ¼ teaspoon kosher salt
- ⅛ teaspoon ground black pepper
- 3 cups loosely packed kale leaves, chopped
- 6 large eggs
- ¾ cup full-fat feta cheese, crumbled
- 2 tablespoons fresh flat-leaf parsley leaves, chopped
- 3 whole-wheat pitas, halved

1. Heat the oil in a large sauté pan over medium heat. Once it is shimmering, add the onions and sauté until softened, about 3 minutes. Add the peppers and garlic, and cook until fragrant, about 4 minutes. Stir in the crushed tomatoes, lentils, cumin, paprika, cayenne, salt, and pepper. Increase the heat to medium-high and bring the mixture to a boil, then reduce the heat to medium-low. Cover the pan and simmer for about 10 minutes , stirring once or twice, until the lentils are very tender and partially melded into the sauce.
2. Stir in the kale, cover, and allow to wilt for 5 minutes. Uncover the pan and stir to combine.
3. Crack 1 egg into a small bowl. Gently pour the egg into the pan along the outer edge. Repeat with the remaining 5 eggs so a circle is formed with the eggs along the outer edge of the pan, leaving at least 2 inches between the eggs. Reduce the heat to low, cover the pan, and cook until the eggs are poached, about 8 minutes. Sprinkle with the feta and parsley.
4. *To serve:* In each of six bowls, spoon 1 cup of the lentil mixture with 1 egg. Serve each with half a pita.
5. *To meal prep:* Place 1 cup of the lentil mixture with 1 egg in each of six individual resealable containers. Let cool, cover, and store for up to 4 days in the refrigerator. To store in the freezer, place in freezer-safe containers; will keep for up to 2 months.

recipe continues 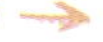

6. *To reheat:* Thaw frozen shakshuka in the refrigerator overnight. To reheat in the microwave, place onto a microwave-safe plate. Heat, uncovered, on high for 1 minute. Let cool for 2 minutes to allow the heat to evenly distribute. To reheat on the stove, place in a small saucepan over medium heat. Cook until the sauce begins to bubble, about 10 minutes. Serve with pita and enjoy warm.

Nutrition Information (per serving): Calories 332; Total Fat 13g; Saturated Fat 5g; Protein 19g; Total Carbohydrates 39g; Fiber 8g; Total Sugars 9g (Includes Added Sugars 0g); Sodium 908mg

Toby's Tip: Swap the lentils for any white bean (like cannellini or Great Northern) or chickpeas. For a heartier base, add diced eggplant to the pan with the onions and let it soften before adding the tomatoes.

Apple-Walnut Cottage Cheese Bowls

At 12 to 13 grams of protein per half-cup serving, cottage cheese is a protein superstar! This bowl is topped with additional protein options, including walnuts and sunflower seeds, for a whopping 17 grams of protein.

PREP TIME 10 min // **COOK TIME** 0 min // **TOTAL TIME** 10 min // **SERVINGS** 4 // **SERVING SIZE** 1 bowl

Meal Prep, One Pot/Pan, 30 Minutes or Less | Vegetarian, Gluten-Free

- 2 cups 2 percent cottage cheese, divided
- 1 medium crisp apple (such as Honeycrisp, Cosmic Crisp, Granny Smith, Fuji), cubed
- ½ cup shelled walnuts, chopped, divided
- ¼ cup unsalted dry-roasted sunflower seeds, divided
- 8 teaspoons pure maple syrup, divided
- ½ teaspoon ground cinnamon, divided

1. In each of four small bowls, spoon ½ cup cottage cheese and top with one-quarter of the apple, 2 tablespoons walnuts, and 1 tablespoon sunflower seeds. Drizzle with 2 teaspoons maple syrup and sprinkle with ⅛ teaspoon cinnamon. Serve immediately.
2. *To meal prep*: Put the cottage cheese and toppings in separate covered containers. Store in the refrigerator for up to four days. When ready to eat, combine ingredients as listed.

Nutrition Information (per serving): Calories 285; Total Fat 15g; Saturated Fat 2g; Protein 17g; Total Carbohydrates 23g; Fiber 3g; Total Sugars 19g (Includes Added Sugars 9g); Sodium 375mg

Toby's Tip: To up your calories and add a few more grams of protein, add a slice of 100 percent whole-wheat bread or whole-grain crackers.

Blueberry-Lemon Chia Seed Pudding

Chia seeds have long been part of health- and plant-forward recipes. Also known as Salba chia and Mexican chia, they are the edible seeds of a flowering plant from the mint family. Besides providing about 6 grams of protein per tablespoon, research shows that these tiny seeds may play a role in the prevention of chronic diseases like heart disease and may potentially help constipation and gastrointestinal-related diseases.

PREP TIME 15 min + overnight // **COOK TIME** 0 min| **TOTAL TIME** 15 min + overnight // **SERVINGS** 4

SERVING SIZE 1 jar

Meal Prep, One Pot/Pan | **Vegan, Vegetarian, Gluten-Free, Dairy-Free**

- 2 cups ultra-filtered milk (13 grams protein per 1 cup serving), divided
- ½ cup chia seeds, divided
- 8 teaspoons honey or agave syrup, divided
- 1 teaspoon lemon zest, divided
- 1 cup vanilla nonfat Greek yogurt, divided
- 1 cup fresh blueberries, divided
- ½ cup unsalted dry-roasted almonds, chopped, divided

1. In each of four (8-ounce) mason jars, stir together ½ cup milk, 2 tablespoons chia seeds, 2 teaspoons honey or agave, and ¼ teaspoon lemon zest.
2. Cover the jars, shake well, and place in the refrigerator until the pudding has solidified, overnight or up to 4 days.
3. *To serve:* Top each portion of pudding with ¼ cup yogurt, ¼ cup blueberries, and 2 tablespoons almonds. Enjoy!
4. *To meal prep:* Store the jars and toppings in separate resealable containers and refrigerate for up to 4 days. Add the toppings just prior to eating.

Nutrition Information (per serving): Calories 317; Total Fat 14g; Saturated Fat 1g; Protein 18g; Total Carbohydrates 33g; Fiber 11g; Total Sugars 18g (Includes Added Sugars 5.75g); Sodium 85mg

Toby's Tip: Be sure to stir well before refrigerating to prevent the chia seeds from clumping at the bottom.

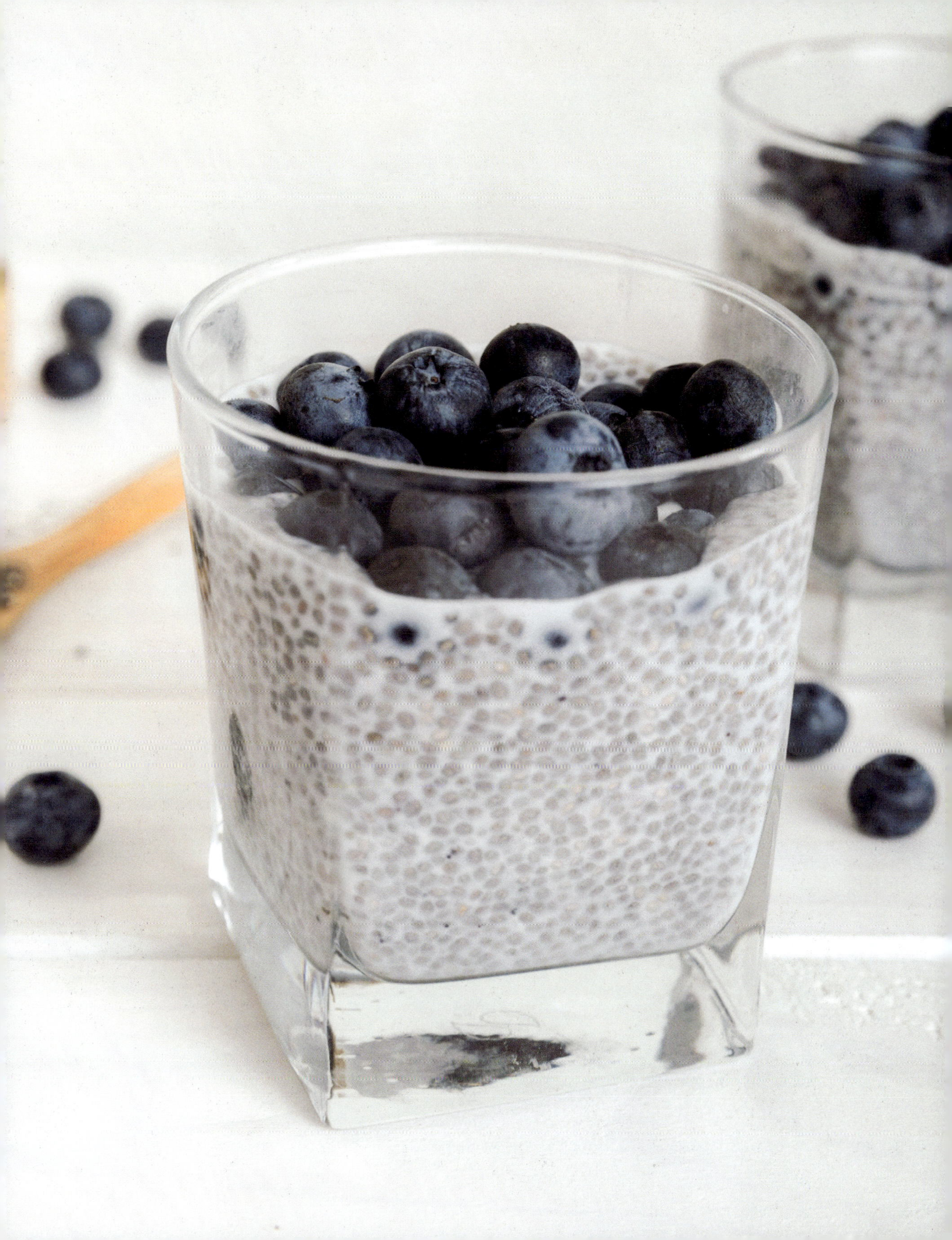

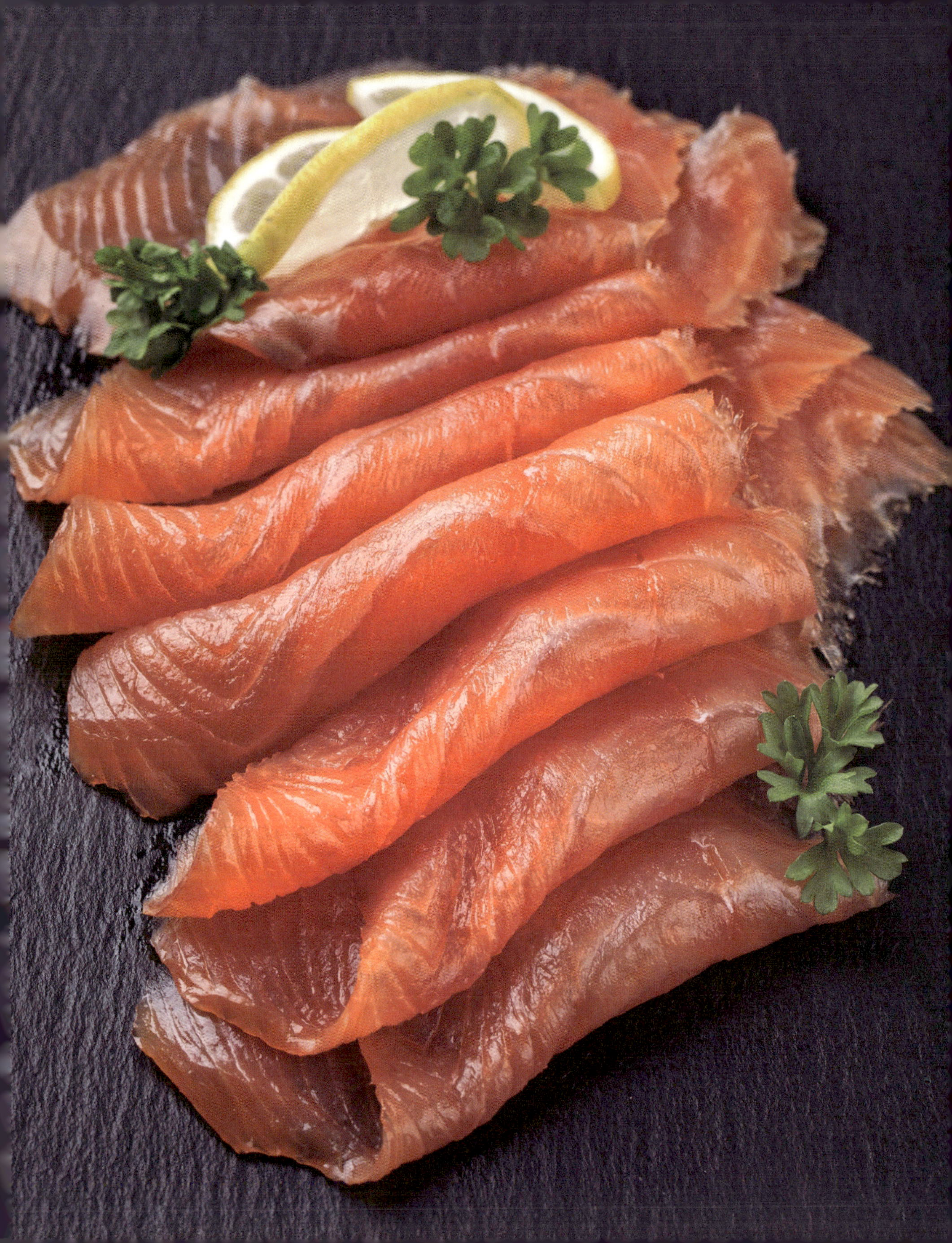

Smoked Salmon and Goat Cheese Toast

An elegant upgrade to your morning meal, this toast combines savory smoked salmon with a tangy and refreshing cucumber and onion topping.

PREP TIME 30 min // **COOK TIME** 0 min // **TOTAL TIME** 30 min // **SERVINGS** 4 // **SERVING SIZE** 1 slice of bread

30 Minutes or Less

- 1 Persian or Kirby (mini) cucumber
- ¼ medium red onion
- 2 teaspoons capers, drained
- 2 tablespoons fresh dill, chopped
- 2 tablespoons red wine vinegar
- ⅛ teaspoon ground black pepper
- ¼ cup extra-virgin olive oil
- 4 slices whole-grain Italian bread, toasted
- 10 ounces smoked salmon
- ¼ cup crumbled full-fat goat cheese

1. Using a mandolin, thinly slice the cucumbers and onions. Place in a small bowl. Add the capers and dill; toss to combine and set aside.
2. In a separate small bowl, whisk together the vinegar and pepper. While whisking briskly, drizzle in the oil until combined. Pour the dressing over the cucumber mixture and toss to combine. Cover the bowl and refrigerate to allow the flavors to meld, for 20 minutes or up to 8 hours.
3. *To serve:* Dip a brush into the dressing and brush over one side of each slice of bread. Add 2½ ounces smoked salmon, ⅓ cup of the cucumber mixture with the dressing, and 1 tablespoon goat cheese. Serve immediately.

Nutrition Information (per serving): Calories 300; Total Fat 20g; Saturated Fat 4g; Protein 18g; Total Carbohydrates 13g; Fiber 3g; Total Sugars 3g (Includes Added Sugars 0g); Sodium 754mg

Toby's Tip: Prepare the cucumber-onion mixture the night before for a quicker morning.

Black Beans and Eggs Breakfast Bowl

Start your day with a protein-packed bean breakfast that's perfect for busy mornings. This easy-to-make dish can be prepped ahead of time, so you can simply heat and eat it during your busy weekday schedule.

PREP TIME 20 min // **COOK TIME** 31 min // **TOTAL TIME** 51 min // **SERVINGS** 4 // **SERVING SIZE** 1 bowl

Meal Prep, Freezer-Friendly | **Vegetarian**

2 tablespoons olive oil, divided

2 cloves garlic, minced

2 jalapeño peppers, seeds and ribs removed, chopped

2 (15.5-ounce) cans low-sodium black beans, with liquid

¼ cup low-sodium vegetable broth or water

1 teaspoon ground cumin

1 teaspoon dried oregano leaves

½ teaspoon chili powder

½ teaspoon kosher salt, divided

4 large eggs

2 tablespoons fresh cilantro leaves, chopped

1 medium yellow onion, cut into ½-inch-thick slices

2 medium green bell peppers, seeds and ribs removed, cut into ½-inch strips

¼ teaspoon ground black pepper

½ cup (3 ounces) Cotija cheese, crumbled

1 avocado, pitted and sliced

1 lime, quartered

1. Heat 1 tablespoon of the oil in a large skillet over medium heat. Once it is shimmering, add the garlic and jalapeños, and cook until fragrant, about 1 minute. Add the black beans with the liquid and stir to combine. Add the vegetable broth or water, cumin, oregano, chili powder, and ¼ teaspoon of the kosher salt; stir to combine. Increase the heat to high and bring the mixture to a boil. Reduce the heat to medium-low and simmer, uncovered, for 15 minutes to reduce the liquid; stir to combine.

2. Crack 1 egg into a small bowl. Gently pour the egg into the pan along the outer edge. Repeat with the remaining 3 eggs, spacing each at least 3 inches apart. Reduce the heat to low, cover the pan, and cook until the eggs are cooked, about 10 minutes. Turn the heat off, sprinkle with the cilantro, and set the skillet aside.

3. Heat the remaining 1 tablespoon of oil in a medium sauté pan over medium heat. Once it is shimmering, add the onion and green peppers, and cook until the vegetables are softened, about 5 minutes. Sprinkle with the remaining ¼ teaspoon of salt and black pepper and toss to combine. Remove the pan from the heat and set aside.

4. *To serve:* In each of four bowls, spoon 1 cup of the bean mixture with 1 egg, spoon ¾ cup of the onion-pepper mixture on the side of the beans, and sprinkle the bowl with 2 tablespoons of Cotija cheese. Place one-quarter of the avocado slices and one-quarter slice of the lime in the bowl and serve warm.

5. *To meal prep:* Place 1 cup of the bean mixture, 1 egg, ¾ cup of the onion-pepper mixture, and 2 tablespoons of the Cotija cheese into each of four resealable containers. Place the quarter slice of lime into the top of each container. Refrigerate for up to 4 days.

6. *To reheat:* Remove the lime quarter from the container and reserve. Transfer to a microwave-safe container or plate and heat on high in the microwave for 1½ minutes. Serve warm with the reserved lime and avocado.

Nutrition Information (per serving): Calories 398; Total Fat 21g; Saturated Fat 6g; Protein 20g; Total Carbohydrates 42g; Fiber 15g; Total Sugars 5g (Includes Added Sugars 0g); Sodium 890mg

Toby's Tip: To add more spice, increase the quantity of chili powder to 1 teaspoon, and drizzle with hot sauce before serving.

Peach Compote Parfaits

No birthday in our family is complete without a fresh batch of compote. While these instructions feature peaches, you can use any combination of fruit you like, such as mango or pineapple.

PREP TIME 20 min // **COOK TIME** 21 min // **TOTAL TIME** 41 min // **SERVINGS** 4 // **SERVING SIZE** 1 parfait

Meal Prep | **Vegetarian, Gluten-Free**

3 cups peach slices, fresh or frozen

¼ cup 100 percent orange juice

1 tablespoon pure maple syrup

1 teaspoon ground cinnamon

½ cup sunflower seed butter

1 teaspoon pure vanilla extract

2 cups plain nonfat Greek yogurt

¼ cup unsalted dry-roasted sunflower seeds, divided

¼ cup unsweetened coconut flakes, divided

1. In a medium saucepan, stir together the peaches, orange juice, maple syrup, and cinnamon. Bring to a boil over high heat. Reduce the heat to medium-low, cover, and cook, stirring occasionally, until the mixture softens and becomes gel-like, about 20 minutes. Remove from heat and set aside to slightly cool, about 15 minutes.
2. In a microwave-safe bowl, stir together the sunflower seed butter and vanilla. Microwave on high until the mixture turns into a liquid, about 30 seconds. Set aside to slightly cool, about 5 minutes.
3. *To serve:* In each of four tall glasses, add ¼ cup Greek yogurt and top with 1 tablespoon of the sunflower seed butter and ¼ cup of the peach compote. Repeat a second layer and then sprinkle with 1 tablespoon each of the sunflower seeds and coconut flakes.
4. *To meal prep:* Cover and refrigerate the parfait cups for up to 4 days.

Nutrition Information (per serving): Calories 401; Total Fat 24g; Saturated Fat 4g; Protein 20g; Total Carbohydrates 32g; Fiber 5g; Total Sugars 23g (Includes Added Sugars 3.5g); Sodium 68mg

Toby's Tip: Use the compote to top the Protein Pancakes on page 113.

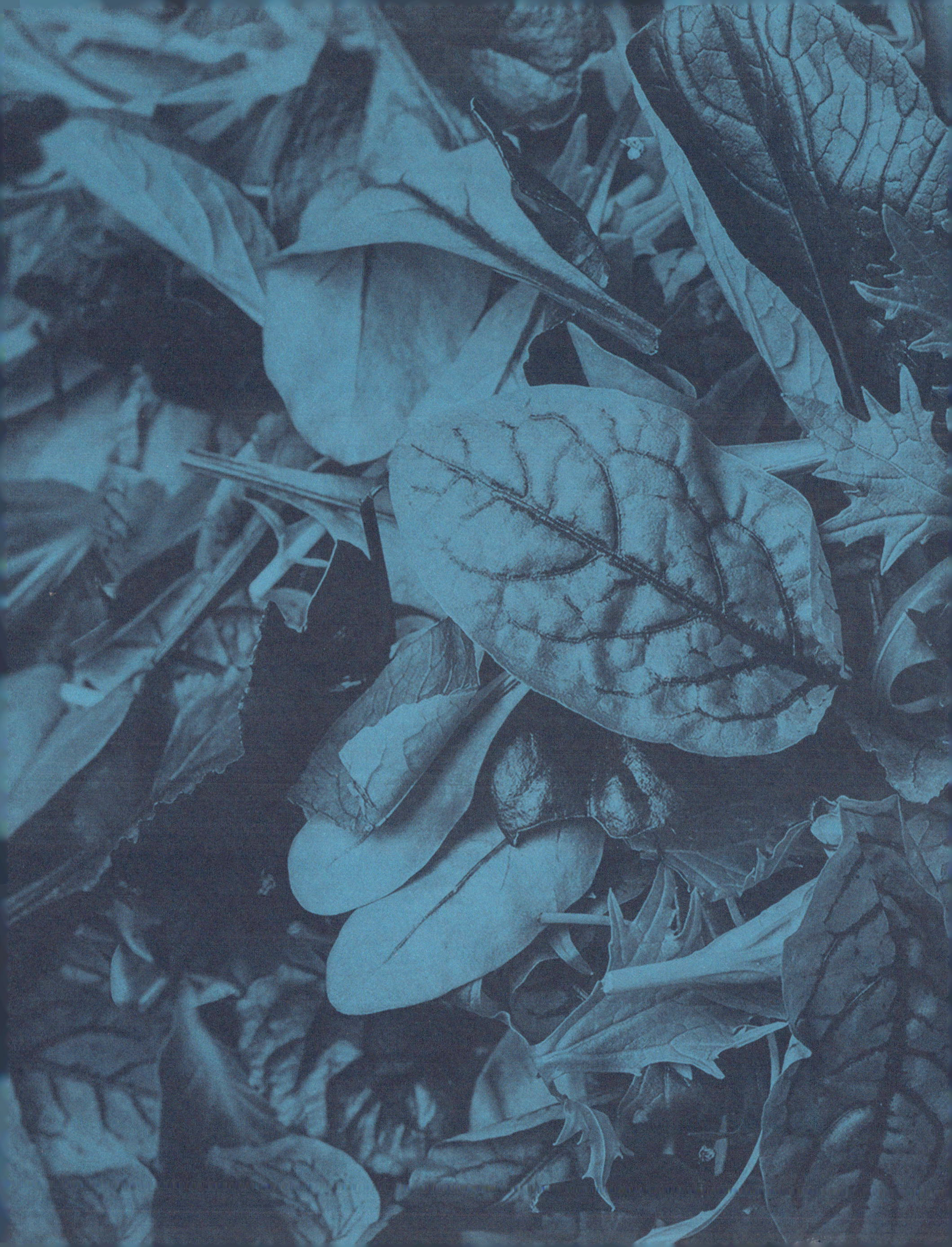

CHAPTER 6

Salads, Sandwiches, and Wraps

Grilled Tofu and Vegetable Salad

A satisfying and crisp salad featuring tender tofu, hearty chickpeas, and a vibrant medley of zucchini, tomatoes, and mushrooms mixed with refreshing romaine.

PREP TIME 40 min // **COOK TIME** 12 min // **TOTAL TIME** 52 min // **SERVINGS** 4

SERVING SIZE 2½ cups salad + 2 tablespoons dressing

Meal Prep | **Vegan, Gluten-Free, Dairy-Free**

- 1 pound extra-firm tofu
- 6 tablespoons balsamic vinegar
- 2 teaspoons Dijon mustard
- ½ teaspoon kosher salt
- ¼ teaspoon ground black pepper
- ¾ cup + 2 tablespoons extra-virgin olive oil, divided
- 1 medium zucchini, sliced lengthwise and then cut into ½-inch half-moons
- 8 ounces button mushrooms, halved
- 1 cup cherry tomatoes
- 4 cups loosely packed romaine lettuce, chopped
- 1 (15.5-ounce) can low-sodium chickpeas, rinsed and drained
- ⅓ cup unsalted dry-roasted sunflower seeds

1. Drain the water from the tofu container. Then wrap the tofu in paper towels or a clean dish towel, and place it on a plate or cutting board. Place a heavy skillet or pan on top to apply pressure and set aside for at least 30 minutes to press out liquid (leave longer for a firmer texture). Cut the tofu into 1-inch cubes.
2. In a small bowl, whisk together the vinegar, mustard, salt, and pepper. While whisking, slowly drizzle ¾ cup of the oil into the mixture until fully incorporated.
3. In a medium bowl, add the zucchini, mushrooms, and tomatoes. Pour over 5 tablespoons of the vinaigrette and toss to evenly coat. Cover the bowl and place in the refrigerator to marinate for at least 20 minutes or up to 2 hours.
4. In a separate medium bowl, add the tofu and 5 tablespoons of the vinaigrette; toss to evenly coat. Cover the bowl and place in the refrigerator to marinate for at least 20 minutes or up to 2 hours.
5. Heat 1 tablespoon of the oil in a medium grill or sauté pan over medium heat. Once it is shimmering, add the vegetables and cook until slightly brown, turning occasionally, about 8 minutes. Transfer the vegetables to a clean bowl.

6. In the same grill or sauté pan, heat the remaining 1 tablespoon of oil over medium heat. Once the oil is shimmering, add the tofu and cook for 2 minutes on each side. Transfer the tofu to a clean bowl.
7. *To serve:* In a large salad bowl, add the romaine lettuce and chickpeas, then the grilled vegetables, and top with the tofu and sunflower seeds. Pour over the remaining vinaigrette and toss to evenly coat. Serve immediately.
8. *To meal prep:* Place 2½ cups of the salad into each of four resealable containers. In four smaller resealable containers, add 2 tablespoons of the dressing. Cover the containers and refrigerate for up to 4 days. Pour the dressing over the salad before eating.

Nutrition Information (per serving): Calories 569; Total Fat 45g; Saturated Fat 5g; Protein 20g; Total Carbohydrates 28g; Fiber 8g; Total Sugars 9g (Includes Added Sugars 0g); Sodium 281mg

Toby's Tip: Swap the tofu with boneless, skinless chicken breast. Cook the chicken, turning at least once, until it reaches an internal temperature of 165°F, about 8 minutes.

Strawberry Shrimp Salad *with* Lemon Basil Vinaigrette

This elegant salad features succulent shrimp and sweet strawberries, brought together by tangy and earthy basil vinaigrette—a perfect choice any time of the year.

PREP TIME 40 min // **COOK TIME** 4 min // **TOTAL TIME** 44 min // **SERVINGS** 4

SERVING SIZE ~2 cups + 2 tablespoons vinaigrette

Meal Prep | **Vegetarian, Gluten-Free**

FOR THE VINAIGRETTE

Juice of 2 lemons

1 teaspoon Dijon mustard

1 clove garlic, minced

½ teaspoon dried basil

½ teaspoon kosher salt

¼ teaspoon ground black pepper

½ cup + 2 tablespoons extra-virgin olive oil, divided

FOR THE SALAD

1 pound large shrimp, peeled and deveined

4 cups loosely packed baby spinach

2 Kirby or mini cucumbers, halved and cut into 1-inch half-moons

1 cup (8 medium) strawberries, hulled and thinly sliced

½ small red onion, cut into ¼-inch strips

⅓ cup (2 ounces) full-fat goat cheese, crumbled

1. In a small bowl, whisk together the lemon juice, mustard, garlic, basil, salt, and pepper. While whisking, slowly drizzle ½ cup of the oil into the mixture until incorporated.
2. Place the shrimp in a medium bowl. Drizzle with ¼ cup of the vinaigrette; toss to combine. Cover the bowl and refrigerate for 20 minutes or up to 2 hours.
3. Heat the remaining 2 tablespoons of oil in a large skillet over medium heat. Once it is shimmering, add the shrimp and cook until they are opaque, about 2 minutes on each side. Transfer the shrimp to a clean bowl.
4. *To serve:* In a large salad bowl, add the spinach, cucumbers, strawberries, onions, and cooked shrimp. Sprinkle with the crumbled goat cheese. Drizzle with the remaining ½ cup vinaigrette and toss to combine. Serve immediately.

5. *To meal prep:* In each of four resealable containers, place ¾ cup spinach, one-quarter of the cucumbers, about 3 ounces of the cooked shrimp, and ¼ each of the strawberries, onions, and goat cheese. In each of four small resealable containers, spoon 2 tablespoons of the vinaigrette; cover and place one inside each of the salad containers. Cover the larger containers and refrigerate for up to 4 days. Pour the dressing over the salad before eating.

Nutrition Information (per serving): Calories 464; Total Fat 38g; Saturated Fat 8g; Protein 27g; Total Carbohydrates 9g; Fiber 2g; Total Sugars 4g (Includes Added Sugars 0g); Sodium 410mg

Toby's Tip: To balance the meal, serve with a small dinner roll.

Peanut-Flavored Slaw *with* Sautéed Chicken

Visually stunning and delicious, purple cabbage is the star of this umami-packed dish. The savory peanut butter dressing and chicken provide nearly 40 grams of protein per serving.

PREP TIME 40 min // **COOK TIME** 8 min // **TOTAL TIME** 48 min // **SERVINGS** 4 // **SERVING SIZE** 1¾ cups

Meal Prep | **Dairy-free**

1 jalapeño pepper, seeds and ribs removed, cut into ⅛-inch dice

1½ tablespoons dark brown sugar

1 tablespoon reduced-sodium soy sauce

Juice of 2 limes, divided

1 teaspoon Dijon mustard

1 pound boneless, skinless chicken breast, cut into bite-size pieces

4 cups loosely packed red cabbage, shredded

2 medium carrots, shredded

1 cup bean sprouts

2 green onions, chopped

¼ cup fresh cilantro leaves, chopped

½ cup water

½ cup smooth peanut butter

1 teaspoon fish sauce

1 teaspoon hot sauce or sriracha-style sauce

1 clove garlic, minced

¼ teaspoon ground ginger

1 tablespoon olive oil

¼ cup unsalted dry-roasted peanuts, chopped

1. In a medium bowl, whisk together the jalapeño, sugar, soy sauce, juice of 1 lime, and mustard. Add the chicken pieces and toss to coat. Cover the bowl and refrigerate for at least 20 minutes or up to 24 hours.
2. Meanwhile, in a large bowl, combine the cabbage, carrots, bean sprouts, onions, and cilantro.
3. In a medium bowl, whisk together the water, peanut butter, juice of the remaining lime, fish sauce, hot sauce, garlic, and ginger. Pour the dressing over the vegetables and toss to evenly coat.
4. Heat the oil in a medium skillet over medium heat. Once it is shimmering, add the chicken, discarding the excess marinade, and cook for about 8 minutes, turning the pieces over halfway through, until browned on both sides. Remove the pan from the heat and set aside to cool for 10 minutes.
5. *To serve:* In a large serving bowl, add the slaw, top with the cooked chicken, and sprinkle with the peanuts. Serve immediately.

6. *To meal prep:* In each of four resealable containers, spoon 1¾ cups salad. Cover and refrigerate for up to 4 days. Serve with the peanuts.

Nutrition Information (per serving): Calories 494; Total Fat 28g; Saturated Fat 5g; Protein 39g; Total Carbohydrates 27g; Fiber 6g; Total Sugars 12g (Includes Added Sugars 4.5g); Sodium 537mg

Toby's Tip: To soften the peanut butter, place in a microwave-safe dish and microwave on high for 30 seconds. Allow to cool for 2 minutes before using.

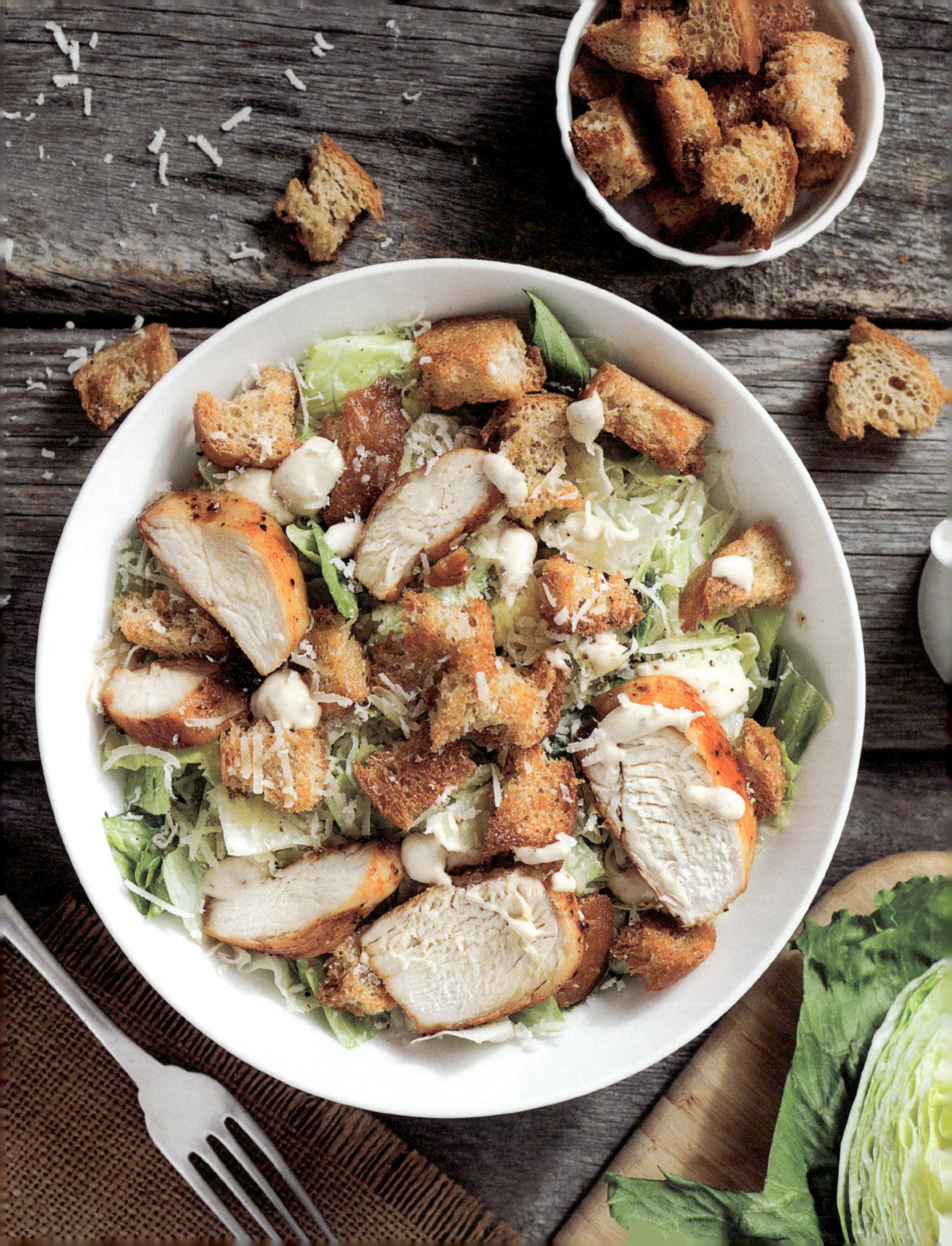

Caesar Salad *with* Chicken Breast

This go-to restaurant dish is a breeze to make at home. Just add your favorite protein! This version features chicken breast marinated in lemon-thyme vinaigrette paired with crispy homemade garlic-herb croutons.

PREP TIME 30 min // **COOK TIME** 18 min // **TOTAL TIME** 48 min // **SERVINGS** 4 // **SERVING SIZE** 2½ cups

Meal Prep

FOR THE CHICKEN

Juice of 1 lemon

¼ cup extra-virgin olive oil, divided

1 clove garlic, minced

1 teaspoon dried thyme

½ teaspoon kosher salt

¼ teaspoon ground black pepper

¾ pound chicken breast

FOR THE GARLIC AND HERB CROUTONS

¼ cup extra-virgin olive oil

½ teaspoon garlic powder

1 teaspoon dried rosemary

1 teaspoon dried parsley

½ teaspoon kosher salt

¼ teaspoon ground black pepper

3 slices country-style white bread, cut into 1-inch cubes

FOR THE CAESAR DRESSING

¼ cup plain nonfat Greek yogurt

2 tablespoons light mayonnaise

2 tablespoons grated Parmesan cheese

2 tablespoons extra-virgin olive oil

1 tablespoon lemon juice

1 teaspoon Dijon mustard

1 teaspoon Worcestershire sauce

⅛ teaspoon garlic powder

⅛ teaspoon ground black pepper

6 cups loosely packed romaine lettuce, chopped

2 tablespoons Parmesan cheese, grated

1. *For the chicken:* In a medium bowl, add the lemon juice, 2 tablespoons of the oil, garlic, thyme, salt, and pepper. Add the chicken and toss to evenly coat. Cover the bowl and place in the refrigerator to marinate for at least 20 minutes or up to 24 hours.
2. Heat the remaining 2 tablespoons of the oil in a large skillet over medium heat. Once it is shimmering, add the chicken breast, shaking off the excess marinade, and cook until the chicken reaches an internal temperature of 145°F, about 4 minutes on each side. Transfer the cooked chicken to a clean plate and allow to slightly cool, about 10 minutes. Discard excess marinade.
3. *For the croutons:* Preheat the oven to 400°F and line a rimmed baking sheet with a silicon mat or parchment paper.

recipe continues 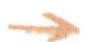

4. In a medium bowl, whisk together the oil, garlic powder, rosemary, parsley, salt, and pepper. Toss the cubed bread into the mixture until the oil is soaked up.
5. Arrange the bread cubes in a single layer on the prepared baking sheet. Bake until browned and toasted, about 10 minutes, tossing halfway through.
6. Remove the baking sheet from the oven and allow to cool for at least 10 minutes. Use a spatula to break up any croutons that may be stuck together.
7. *For the dressing:* In a small bowl, whisk together the yogurt, mayonnaise, Parmesan, oil, lemon juice, mustard, Worcestershire, garlic powder, and pepper.
8. *To serve:* Place the romaine into a large serving bowl. Top with the cooked chicken, croutons, and cheese. Drizzle with the dressing and toss to evenly coat. Serve immediately.
9. *To meal prep:* In each of four resealable containers, place 1½ cups romaine lettuce, about 2 ounces of chicken, about ½ cup of croutons, and 1 tablespoon of Parmesan. In each of four small containers, spoon 2 tablespoons of the dressing. Cover the dressing containers and place one inside each of the salad containers or on the side. Cover the large salad containers and refrigerate for up to 4 days. Dress the salad just before serving.

Nutrition Information (per serving): Calories 465; Total Fat 32g; Saturated Fat 5g; Protein 30g; Total Carbohydrates 20g; Fiber 2g; Total Sugars 4g (Includes Added Sugars 0g); Sodium 600mg

Toby's Tip: If you choose to use extra-virgin olive oil, make sure it is a high-quality extra-virgin olive oil, which has a higher smoke point and can be used stovetop, or if you do not want to spend the money on high-quality EVOO, then use regular olive oil.

Taco Salad *with* Ground Beef and Cilantro-Lime Vinaigrette

This healthful twist on a taco is a deconstructed salad that features ground beef and black beans, along with crushed tortilla chips for extra crunch.

PREP TIME 30 min // **COOK TIME** 8 min // **TOTAL TIME** 38 min // **SERVINGS** 4

SERVING SIZE 2¼ cups + 2 tablespoons dressing

Meal Prep

FOR THE GROUND BEEF

1 teaspoon chili powder

1 teaspoon ground cumin

½ teaspoon smoked paprika

¼ teaspoon dried oregano

½ teaspoon kosher salt

¼ teaspoon garlic powder

¼ teaspoon onion powder

2 tablespoons olive oil

12 ounces ground beef (at least 90 percent lean)

FOR THE CILANTRO-LIME DRESSING

3 tablespoons lime juice

2 tablespoons fresh cilantro leaves, chopped

½ teaspoon ground cumin

½ teaspoon kosher salt

¼ teaspoon garlic powder

¼ teaspoon ground black pepper

6 tablespoons extra-virgin olive oil

FOR THE SALAD

4 cups loosely packed romaine lettuce, shredded

1 cup low-sodium pinto beans, rinsed and drained

½ cup (2 ounces) black olives, chopped, pitted

½ cup (1 ounce) tortilla chips, crushed

½ cup shredded reduced-fat Mexican cheese blend

2 plum tomatoes, diced

2 scallions, thinly sliced, greens and whites

1. *For the ground beef:* In a small bowl, mix the chili powder, cumin, smoked paprika, oregano, salt, garlic powder, and onion powder.
2. Heat the oil in a medium skillet over medium heat. Once it is shimmering, add the ground beef and sprinkle with the spice mixture. Cook the ground beef, breaking up any large pieces with a wooden spoon, until cooked through, about 8 minutes. Set aside to cool for at least 10 minutes.
3. *For the Cilantro-Lime Dressing:* In a small bowl, whisk together the lime juice, cilantro, cumin, salt, garlic powder, and pepper. Whisking continuously, slowly drizzle in the oil until incorporated.

recipe continues 

4. *To serve:* In a large serving bowl, add the lettuce, ground beef, beans, olives, tortilla chips, cheese, tomatoes, and scallions. Drizzle with the dressing and toss to evenly coat. Serve immediately.

5. *To meal prep*: In each of four resealable containers, place 2¼ cups of the salad. In each of four small resealable containers, spoon 2 tablespoons of the dressing. Cover containers and refrigerate for up to 4 days. Drizzle the dressing on the salad before serving.

Nutrition Information (per serving): Calories 564; Total Fat 43g; Saturated Fat 9g; Protein 25g; Total Carbohydrates 21g; Fiber 5g; Total Sugars 3g (Includes Added Sugars 0g); Sodium 767mg

Toby's Tip: For a creative spin on this dish, swap the ground beef for ground lamb, turkey, or chicken.

Smashed Chickpea Dill Sandwich

This Mediterranean-inspired sandwich filling is made with hearty chickpeas and sesame seed paste (AKA tahini) and complemented with dill, parsley, and tangy lemon juice. Serve the sandwich with a small green salad or pita chips.

PREP TIME 15 min // **COOK TIME** 0 min // **TOTAL TIME** 15 min // **SERVINGS** 4 // **SERVING SIZE** 1 sandwich

Meal Prep, 30 Minutes or Less | Vegetarian

- 1 (15.5-ounce) can low-sodium chickpeas, rinsed and drained
- 2 tablespoons extra-virgin olive oil
- 2 tablespoons tahini (sesame seed paste)
- 1 teaspoon Dijon mustard
- 2 tablespoons fresh dill, chopped
- 2 tablespoons fresh flat-leaf parsley leaves, chopped
- 1 tablespoon lemon juice
- 1 tablespoon capers, drained
- 1 tablespoon unsalted dry-roasted sesame seeds
- 1 scallion, whites and greens, chopped
- ½ teaspoon kosher salt
- ¼ teaspoon ground black pepper
- 8 slices multigrain bread, toasted
- 8 romaine lettuce leaves
- 4 slices reduced-fat Swiss cheese
- 2 plum tomatoes, thinly sliced

1. In a medium bowl, add the chickpeas, oil, tahini, and mustard. Using a potato masher, roughly mash the chickpeas. Add the dill, parsley, lemon juice, capers, sesame seeds, scallions, salt, and pepper; mix well.
2. On each of 4 slices of bread, place 2 lettuce leaves, 1 slice cheese, and several slices of tomato; top with a heaping ⅓ cup of the chickpea mash. Cover with the remaining slices of bread and gently press down to create a sandwich. Slice each sandwich in half and serve.
3. *To meal prep:* In each of four large resealable containers, separate the sandwich ingredients into separate containers or containers with compartments as an assembled sandwich will get soggy. Cover and refrigerate for up to 4 days. Assemble the sandwich before eating.

Nutrition Information (per serving): Calories 395; Total Fat 16g; Saturated Fat 4g; Protein 22g; Total Carbohydrates 49g; Fiber 14g; Total Sugars 9g (Includes Added Sugars 0g); Sodium 758mg

Toby's Tip: Tahini can add a slightly bitter taste to the chickpea mixture; omit it if you prefer.

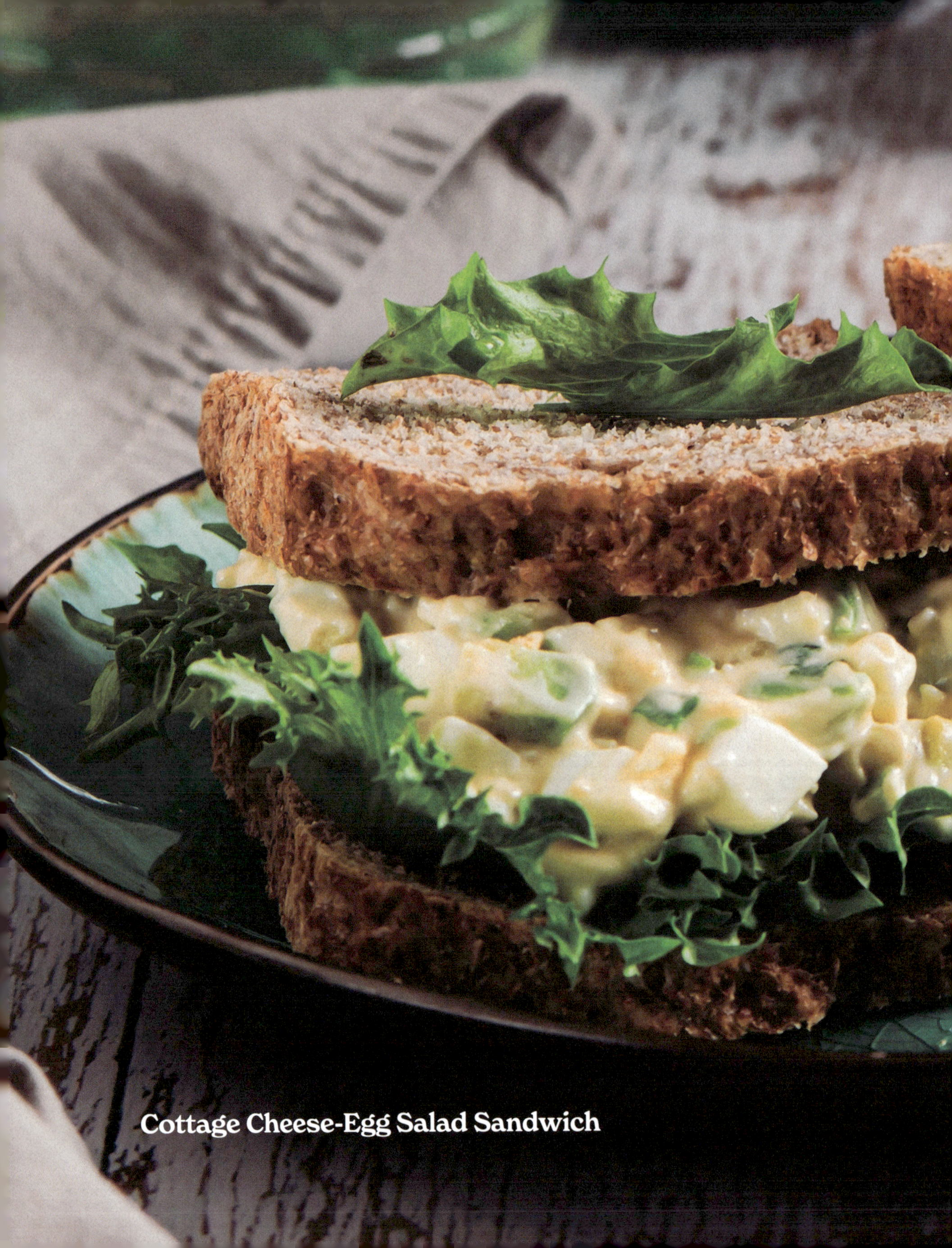

Cottage Cheese-Egg Salad Sandwich

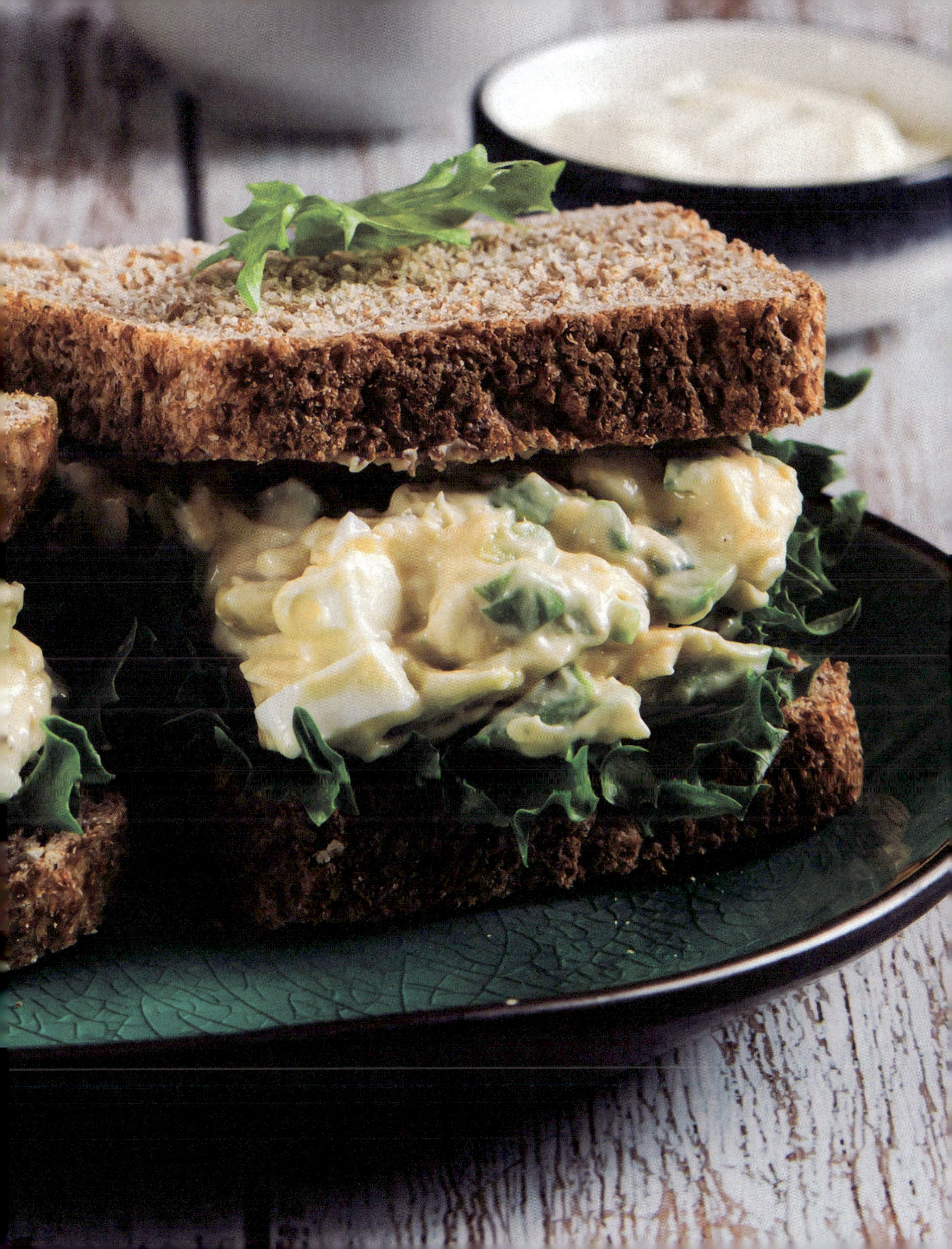

Cottage Cheese-Egg Salad Sandwich

In this sandwich, eggs complemented by creamy, nutritious cottage cheese to deliver a quick, high-protein meal. Serve with a cool cucumber salad or slaw on the side.

PREP TIME 20 min // **COOK TIME** 3 min // **TOTAL TIME** 23 min // **SERVINGS** 4 // **SERVING SIZE** 1 sandwich

Meal Prep, 30 Minutes or Less | **Vegetarian**

2 large eggs

1 cup low-fat 1 percent cottage cheese

1 tablespoon fresh chives, finely chopped

1 tablespoon lemon juice

1 teaspoon smoked paprika

1 teaspoon Dijon mustard

¼ teaspoon kosher salt

¼ teaspoon ground black pepper

1 cup microgreens of choice, loosely packed

8 slices whole-grain bread, toasted

1. Place the eggs in a medium saucepan and cover with cold water. Place the saucepan over high heat and bring the water to a boil; cook for 3 minutes. Remove the saucepan from the heat, cover, and allow to stand for 15 minutes. Drain, then run cold water over the eggs until completely cool, about 10 minutes. Once they have cooled, peel the eggs.
2. In a medium bowl, using a potato masher, mash the eggs, and cottage cheese together; stir until combined. Stir in the parsley, chives, lemon juice, paprika, mustard, salt, and pepper.
3. On each of 4 slices of bread, place ¼ cup of the microgreens and ½ cup of the egg-cottage cheese mixture. Cover each sandwich with the remaining bread slices and gently press down to make a sandwich. Slice each sandwich in half; serve immediately.
4. *To meal prep*: In each of four containers, spoon ½ cup of the egg-cottage cheese mixture. In each of four separate containers, place the remaining ingredients. Store up to 4 days. Assemble the sandwich before eating.

Nutrition Information (per serving): Calories 350; Total Fat 12g; Saturated Fat 3.5g; Protein 20g; Total Carbohydrates 42g; Fiber 7g; Total Sugars 6g (Includes Added Sugars 0g); Sodium 780mg

Toby's Tip: Hard-boil a few extra eggs so you have a protein-filled snack readily available in your refrigerator.

Chopped Salad *with* Chickpeas and Tuna

Finely chopped vegetables, earthy chickpeas, and robustly flavored tuna come together in this bright, satisfying dish, dressed simply with lemon and olive oil dressing.

PREP TIME 20 min // **COOK TIME** 0 min // **TOTAL TIME** 20 min // **SERVINGS** 4 // **SERVING SIZE** ~2 cups

Meal Prep, 30 Minutes or Less | **Vegetarian, Gluten-Free**

- 2 (5-ounce) cans albacore tuna packed in water, drained
- 1 (15.5-ounce) can low-sodium chickpeas, rinsed and drained
- ½ English or hothouse cucumber, chopped
- 2 plum tomatoes, chopped
- 1 yellow or orange medium bell pepper, seeds and ribs removed, chopped
- ¼ small red onion, chopped
- 2 tablespoons fresh flat-leaf parsley leaves, chopped
- Juice of 1 lemon
- 2 tablespoons extra-virgin olive oil
- ¼ teaspoon kosher salt
- ¼ teaspoon ground black pepper
- ½ cup full-fat feta cheese

1. Place the tuna in a large bowl. Using a fork, break the tuna into bite-size pieces. Add the chickpeas, cucumber, tomato, bell pepper, onion, and parsley; toss to combine.
2. Add the lemon juice, oil, salt, and black pepper; toss to evenly coat. Sprinkle with the feta cheese. Serve immediately.
3. *To meal prep:* In each of four resealable containers, spoon ~2 cups of the salad. Cover and refrigerate for up to 4 days.

Nutrition Information (per serving): Calories 306; Total Fat 15g; Saturated Fat 4g; Protein 25g; Total Carbohydrates 21g; Fiber 6g; Total Sugars 7g (Includes Added Sugars 0g); Sodium 789mg

Toby's Tip: If you're a lemon lover, use the juice from 1 whole lemon.

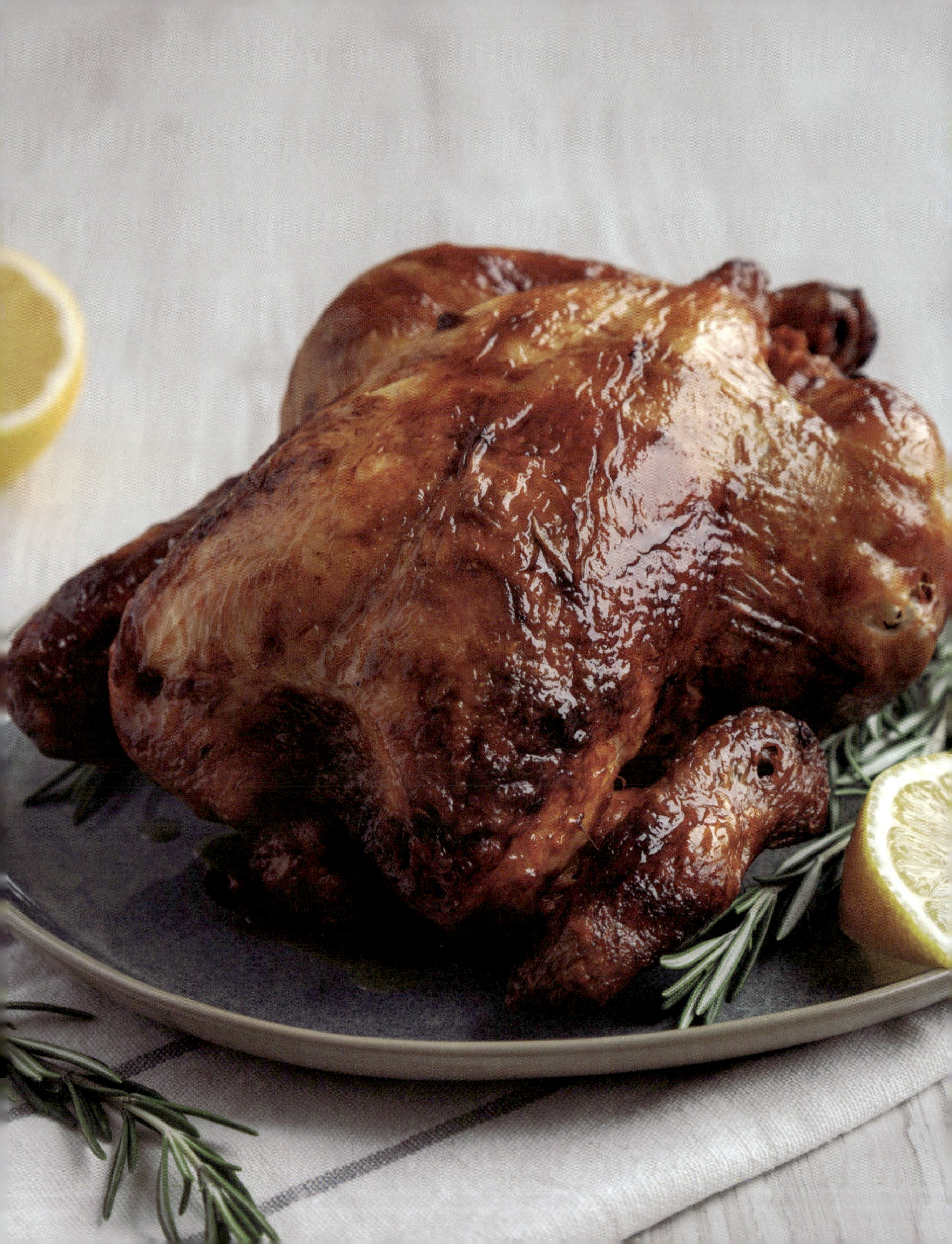

Rotisserie Chicken Wrap *with* Homemade Ranch Dressing

Short on time? Grab a rotisserie chicken to speed things up! Mix it with some homemade light ranch dressing, roll it into a wrap, and serve with your choice of roasted potato wedges or a green salad.

PREP TIME 20 min // **COOK TIME** 0 min // **TOTAL TIME** 20 min // **SERVINGS** 4 // **SERVING SIZE** 1 wrap

Meal Prep, 30 Minutes or Less

FOR THE RANCH DRESSING

¼ cup low-fat buttermilk

3 tablespoons plain reduced-fat (2 percent) Greek yogurt

3 tablespoons light mayonnaise

1 tablespoon fresh flat-leaf parsley leaves, finely chopped

1 tablespoon fresh chives, finely chopped

1 tablespoon lemon juice

1 garlic clove, crushed

¼ teaspoon kosher salt

¼ teaspoon ground black pepper

⅛ teaspoon cayenne pepper

⅛ teaspoon smoked paprika

FOR THE WRAP

2 cups (10 ounces) packed rotisserie chicken without skin, or grilled boneless, skinless chicken breast, shredded

½ cup reduced-fat pepperjack or cheddar cheese

½ cup Ranch Dressing (see recipe)

1 medium scallion, greens and whites, chopped

⅛ teaspoon ground black pepper

1 avocado, pitted and sliced

4 whole-wheat tortillas

1. *For the dressing:* In a blender, combine buttermilk, Greek yogurt, mayonnaise, parsley, chives, lemon juice, garlic, salt, pepper, cayenne, and smoked paprika. Blend on high speed until smooth.
2. Place the dressing in a small container, cover, and place in the refrigerator for at least 30 minutes to chill before using.
3. *For the wrap:* In a medium bowl, add the chicken, cheese, dressing, scallions, and pepper. Mix well.
4. *To serve:* Place each of 4 wraps on a flat work surface. Divide the avocado equally among the wraps and, using a fork, gently mash. Add ½ cup of the chicken mixture to the center of each tortilla. Close the wraps by folding each side toward the center, folding the rounded end up over the filling, and then rolling up to form a cylinder. Enjoy!

recipe continues

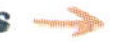

5. *To meal prep:* Tightly cover each wrap in plastic wrap or aluminum foil. Store in the refrigerator for up to 4 days. Best if eaten within 1 day. Ideally, store the chicken salad and wraps separately, and roll together before eating.

Nutrition Information (per serving): Calories 439; Total Fat 22g; Saturated Fat 6g; Protein 31g; Total Carbohydrates 33g; Fiber 8g; Total Sugars 2g (Includes Added Sugars 0g); Sodium 31mg

Toby's Tip: To cut back on the heat, omit the cayenne. To add even more heat, use up to ¼ teaspoon of cayenne.

Turkey Pesto Panini

This panini comes in at over 600 calories, mainly due to the unsaturated fat in the pesto sauce. If you're someone who needs higher calories, this is a perfect portion. If you take in between 1,600 to 1,800 calories per day, opt for half a portion, which still provides 19 grams of protein.

PREP TIME 20 min // **COOK TIME** 5 min // **TOTAL TIME** 25 min // **SERVINGS** 4 // **SERVING SIZE** 1 panini

30 Minutes or Less

FOR THE PESTO

3 tablespoons pine nuts

1 tablespoon Parmesan cheese, grated

1 tablespoon fresh lemon juice

1 clove garlic, crushed

¼ teaspoon kosher salt

⅛ teaspoon ground black pepper

1 cup packed fresh basil leaves

½ cup extra-virgin olive oil

FOR THE PANINI

8 slices Italian whole-grain bread

12 ounces low-sodium deli turkey slices

8 slices Provolone cheese

1 plum tomato, thinly sliced

Nonstick cooking spray

1. *For the pesto:* In a blender or food processor, add the pine nuts, Parmesan, lemon juice, garlic, salt, and black pepper; pulse until well combined. Add the basil leaves and continue pulsing until incorporated. With the motor running, gradually drizzle in the oil and continue pulsing until a paste forms.
2. Transfer the pesto to a small bowl. Cover and refrigerate for up to 4 days.
3. *For the panini:* Arrange 4 bread slices side by side on a flat work surface. Spread about 2 tablespoons of pesto onto each slice of bread. Top with 3 ounces turkey, 2 slices cheese, and a few tomato slices. Cover each with the remaining bread slices to make a sandwich.
4. Coat a grill pan or griddle with nonstick cooking spray and place over medium-low heat. Once the oil is shimmering, place 2 sandwiches and weigh them down with a clean pan. Cook until the cheese begins to melt and the bread has browned, 2 to 3 minutes on each side. Repeat for the remaining sandwiches. Serve warm.

Nutrition Information (per serving): Calories 642; Total Fat 43g; Saturated Fat 10g; Protein 38g; Total Carbohydrates 29g; Fiber 7g; Total Sugars 8g (Includes Added Sugars 0g); Sodium 1,221mg

Toby's Tip: Low-sodium deli meats are typically located behind the deli counter, so ask for them there.

Salmon Salad Stuffed Pita

This salmon salad is made with fresh salmon tossed with a lighter mayo-based dressing. Pair with mandarins or an orange on the side to complete the meal.

PREP TIME 15 min // **COOK TIME** 12 min // **TOTAL TIME** 27 min // **SERVINGS** 4 // **SERVING SIZE** 2 pita halves

Meal Prep, One Pot/Pan, 30 Minutes or Less | Vegetarian

Cooking spray

8 ounces fresh salmon, about 1½ inches thick

⅜ teaspoon kosher salt, divided

⅜ teaspoon ground black pepper, divided

1 stalk of celery, chopped

¼ medium red onion, chopped

2 tablespoons light mayonnaise

2 tablespoons plain nonfat Greek yogurt

1 tablespoon capers, drained

1 tablespoon lemon juice

1 teaspoon ground tarragon

⅛ teaspoon cayenne

4 (8-inch) whole-wheat pitas, halved

2 Kirby or mini cucumbers, cut into ¼-inch strips

2 plum tomatoes, cut into ¼-inch strips

1 cup sprouts of choice

Nutrition Information (per serving): Calories 307; Total Fat 11g; Saturated Fat 2g; Protein 20g; Total Carbohydrates 33g; Fiber 7g; Total Sugars 5g (Includes Added Sugars 0g); Sodium 596mg

1. Preheat the oven to 425°F. Coat a baking sheet with nonstick cooking spray.
2. Sprinkle both sides of the salmon with ⅛ teaspoon each of the salt and pepper. Place on the prepared baking sheet. Bake in the preheated oven until the internal temperature of the salmon reaches 145°F, about 12 minutes. Remove the baking sheet from the oven and allow to cool for 10 minutes. Discard the skin from the salmon.
3. While the salmon is cooking, in a medium bowl, mix together the celery, onion, mayonnaise, yogurt, capers, lemon juice, tarragon, cayenne, and remaining ¼ teaspoon each of the salt and pepper. Add the cooled salmon and, using the tines of a fork, separate the salmon into small pieces. Cover the bowl and refrigerate for at least 20 minutes or up to 2 hours to allow the flavors to meld.
4. Gently open up the pita halves and fill with several slices each of the cucumber and tomato and 2 tablespoons of the sprouts. Add ¼ cup of the salmon salad. Serve immediately.
5. *To meal prep:* In each of four containers, spoon ¼ cup of the salmon salad. In each of four separate containers, pack the remaining ingredients. Cover and refrigerate for up to 3 days. Assemble the sandwich before eating.

Toby's Tip: To add 6 grams of protein per serving, make this using 12 ounces of salmon.

Sirloin Beef Subs *with* Sautéed Peppers and Onions

Pile on the flavor with these lean beef subs, loaded with peppers, onions, and a kick of spicy aioli. It's a satisfying meal for any crowd, delivering a powerful 35 grams of protein per serving.

PREP TIME 40 min | **COOK TIME** 14 min | **TOTAL TIME** 54 min | **SERVINGS** 4 | **SERVING SIZE** 1 sub

FOR THE BEEF

¼ cup olive oil, divided

¼ cup balsamic vinegar

2 tablespoons reduced-sodium soy sauce

1 tablespoon Worcestershire sauce

1 clove garlic, minced

1 teaspoon dried oregano

1 teaspoon Dijon mustard

⅛ teaspoon ground black pepper

1 pound top sirloin steak, cut into ¾-inch slices

FOR THE PEPPERS AND ONIONS

1 tablespoon olive oil

1 red bell pepper, seeds and ribs removed, cut into ½-inch slices

1 medium yellow onion, cut into ½-inch slices

½ teaspoon dried rosemary

¼ teaspoon kosher salt

⅛ teaspoon ground black pepper

FOR CHIPOTLE AIOLI

¼ cup light mayonnaise

1 chipotle pepper in adobo sauce, finely chopped

1 teaspoon adobo sauce (from the can of chipotle peppers)

1 clove garlic, minced

1 teaspoon lime juice

⅛ teaspoon kosher salt

FOR THE SUBS

4 long potato, sub, or hoagle rolls

4 slices [illegible] Provolone cheese

1. *For the beef:* In a medium bowl, whisk together 2 tablespoons of oil and the balsamic vinegar, soy sauce, Worcestershire sauce, garlic, oregano, mustard, and pepper. Add the steak pieces and toss to evenly coat. Cover the bowl and place in the refrigerator to marinate for at least 20 minutes or up to 24 hours.

2. *For the peppers and onions:* Heat 1 tablespoon of oil in a large skillet over medium heat. Once it is shimmering, add the peppers and onions, and toss to combine. Add the rosemary, salt, and pepper, and toss to combine. Cook until the peppers and onions have softened, 6 to 8 minutes. Remove the skillet from the heat and allow to slightly cool.

3. *For the chipotle aioli:* In a small bowl, whisk together the mayonnaise, chipotle pepper, adobo sauce, garlic, lime juice, and salt.

recipe continues 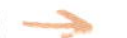

4. *To cook the beef:* Heat the remaining 2 tablespoons of oil in the same skillet over medium heat. Once it is shimmering, add the beef, shaking off the excess marinade, and cook until the internal temperature of the beef reaches 145°F, about 3 minutes on each side. Transfer the beef to a clean plate. Discard excess marinade.
5. *To serve:* In each of 4 rolls, spoon 1 tablespoon chipotle aioli and fold in 1 slice of cheese. Spoon one-quarter of the beef and top with one-quarter of the pepper and onion mixture. Serve warm.

Nutrition Information (per serving): Calories 642; Total Fat 38g; Saturated Fat 11g; Protein 35g; Total Carbohydrates 35g; Fiber 2g; Total Sugars 11g (Includes Added Sugars 5g); Sodium 852mg

Toby's Tip: Swap the sirloin steak for a tenderloin.

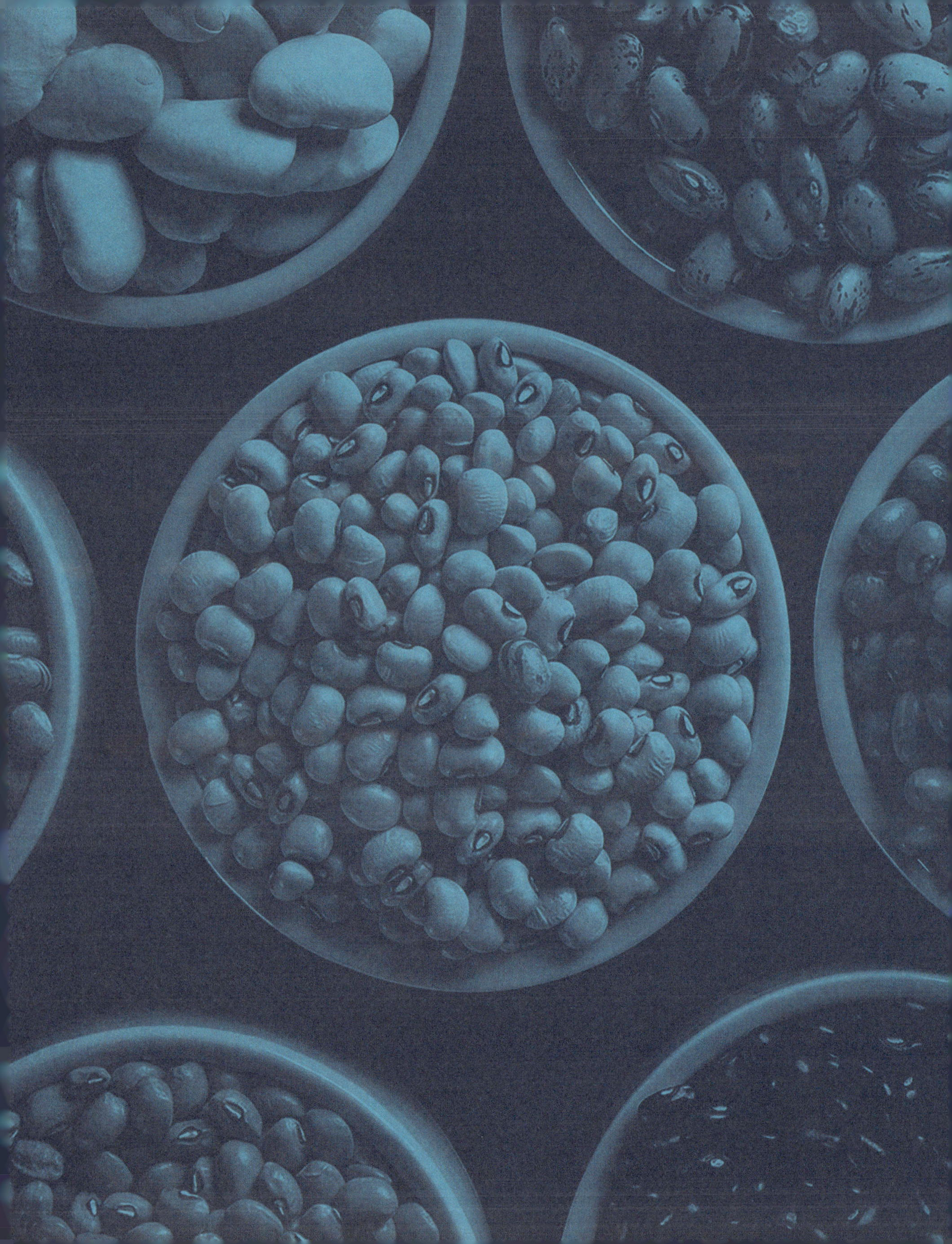

CHAPTER 7

Plant-Based Mains

Lentil Stew

Lentils are an underappreciated pulse that is chock-full of not only protein but also fiber, iron, folate, and potassium. The addition of the peas and flax boost the protein in this plant-only dish to 21 grams.

PREP TIME 20 min // **COOK TIME** 40 min // **TOTAL TIME** 1 hour // **SERVINGS** 4 // **SERVING SIZE** 2 cups

Meal Prep, Freezer-Friendly, One Pot/Pan | Vegan, Vegetarian, Dairy-Free

- 2 tablespoons olive oil
- 1 medium yellow onion, chopped
- 2 cloves garlic, minced
- 2 stalks celery, chopped
- 2 medium carrots, peeled and chopped
- 2 medium russet potatoes, peeled and cut into 1½-inch chunks
- 2 cups low-sodium vegetable broth
- 2 (15.5-ounce) cans brown lentils, rinsed and drained
- 1 (15-ounce) can crushed tomatoes
- 1½ cups frozen peas
- 2 tablespoons ground flaxseed
- 1 tablespoon apple cider vinegar
- 4 bay leaves
- 2 teaspoons smoked paprika
- 1 teaspoon ground cumin
- 1 teaspoon liquid honey
- 3 cups loosely packed kale leaves, chopped
- ½ teaspoon kosher salt
- ¼ teaspoon ground black pepper

1. Heat the oil in a large pot over medium heat. Once the oil is shimmering, add the onions and garlic, and cook until the onions are translucent and garlic is fragrant, about 3 minutes. Add the celery and carrots, and cook until the vegetables have softened, about 5 minutes. Add the potatoes and cook until they are slightly softened, about 5 minutes.
2. Add the broth, lentils, crushed tomatoes, peas, flaxseed, vinegar, bay leaves, paprika, cumin, and honey; stir to combine. Increase the heat to high and bring the mixture to a boil, then reduce the heat to medium-low and simmer, uncovered, until only a few inches of liquid remain and the mixture has thickened, about 25 minutes. Stir in the kale and cook until wilted, about 2 minutes. Stir in the salt and pepper. Discard the bay leaves.
3. *To serve*: Spoon 2 cups of the stew into each of four shallow bowls. Enjoy warm.
4. *To meal prep:* In each of four resealable containers, spoon 2 cups of the stew. Cover and place in the freezer for up to 2 months or in the refrigerator for up to 4 days. To defrost, transfer to the refrigerator at least 24 hours before using.

5. *To reheat*: Transfer the stew to a microwave-safe dish and reheat until the internal temperature is 165°F. Allow to stand for 2 minutes before serving. Alternatively, frozen or refrigerated stew can be reheated stovetop in a shallow saucepan until it reaches a rapid boil, about 10 minutes.

Nutrition Information (per serving): Calories 451; Total Fat 9g; Saturated Fat 1g; Protein 21g; Total Carbohydrates 77g; Fiber 16g; Total Sugars 14g (Includes Added Sugars 1.5g); Sodium 967mg

Toby's Tip: Swap shelled edamame for the peas.

Sheet Pan Spicy Tofu and Vegetables

This is a delicious, well-balanced one-pan meal with tofu, beans, and roasted veggies. The spices deliver a perfect balance of warmth and paprika-infused heat.

PREP TIME 35 min // **COOK TIME** 30 min // **TOTAL TIME** 1 hour, 5 min // **SERVINGS** 4 // **SERVING SIZE** 2 cups

Meal Prep, Freezer-Friendly | Vegan, Vegetarian, Dairy-Free

FOR THE TOFU

1 pound extra-firm tofu

2 tablespoons extra-virgin olive oil

2 teaspoons all-purpose flour

1 teaspoon ground paprika

1 teaspoon ground coriander

1 teaspoon ground cumin

1 teaspoon ground oregano

¼ teaspoon kosher salt

FOR THE VEGETABLES

¼ cup extra-virgin olive oil

2 teaspoons ground paprika

2 teaspoons ground coriander

2 teaspoons ground cumin

2 teaspoons dried parsley

¼ teaspoon kosher salt

1 medium red onion, cut into bite-size chunks

2 red bell peppers, seeds and ribs removed, cut into 1-inch strips

2 cups bite-size broccoli florets

2 cups bite-size cauliflower florets

1 medium sweet potato, peeled and cut into 2-inch chunks

1 (15.5-ounce) can low-sodium kidney beans, rinsed and drained

1. Preheat the oven to 400°F. Line two rimmed baking sheets with parchment paper or silicone liner.
2. *For the tofu:* Wrap the tofu in paper towels or a clean dish towel, and place it on a plate or cutting board. Put a heavy skillet or pan on top to apply pressure and leave it for at least 30 minutes (longer for a firmer texture). Cut the tofu into 1-inch cubes.
3. In a medium bowl, whisk together the oil, flour, paprika, coriander, cumin, oregano, and salt. Add the tofu chunks and toss to evenly coat. Arrange the tofu in a single layer on the center of the prepared baking sheet.
4. *For the vegetables:* In a large bowl, whisk together the oil, paprika, coriander, cumin, parsley, and salt. Add the onion, red peppers, broccoli, cauliflower, and sweet potatoes, and toss to evenly coat. Arrange the vegetables in a single layer on the remaining empty areas of the prepared baking sheets. Sprinkle the beans over the vegetables.
5. Place the baking sheets in the preheated oven and cook until browned, 25 to 30 minutes, turning halfway through.

6. *To serve:* On each of four plates, spoon 2 cups of the vegetables and tofu. Serve warm.
7. *To meal prep:* In each of four resealable containers, spoon 2 cups of the vegetables and tofu. Cover and refrigerate for up to 4 days.
8. *To reheat:* Transfer to a microwave-safe plate and microwave on high for 1½ minutes. Allow to stand for 2 minutes to let the heat distribute evenly before serving.

Nutrition Information (per serving): Calories 425; Total Fat 22g; Saturated Fat 2g; Protein 19g; Total Carbohydrates 40g; Fiber 10g; Total Sugars 10g (Includes Added Sugars 0g); Sodium 366mg

Toby's Tip: Although you don't have to weigh down extra-firm tofu before roasting, I find the tofu has a better texture when doing so.

Tofu and Vegetable Stir-Fry over Almondy Soba Noodles

This dish features earthy soba noodles with a colorful mix of stir-fried carrots, shiitake mushrooms, and bok choy, all tossed in a savory almond butter sauce.

PREP TIME 50 min // **COOK TIME** 23 min // **TOTAL TIME** 1 hour, 13 min // **SERVINGS** 6

SERVING SIZE 1⅔ cups

Meal Prep, Freezer-Friendly | **Vegan, Vegetarian, Gluten-Free, Dairy-Free**

1 pound extra-firm tofu

¼ cup extra-virgin olive oil, divided

1 tablespoon reduced-sodium soy sauce

1 tablespoon apple cider vinegar

8 ounces gluten-free dried soba or buckwheat noodles

½ cup warm water

⅓ cup unsalted almond butter

Juice of 1 lemon

½ teaspoon kosher salt

2 tablespoons olive oil

2 medium carrots, peeled and cut into 1-inch rounds

3½ ounces shiitake or cremini mushrooms, thinly sliced

1 green onion, whites and greens, thinly sliced

1 medium head bok choy, leaves separated and roughly chopped

¼ cup fresh cilantro leaves, chopped

¼ cup unsalted dry-roasted almonds, chopped

1. *For the tofu:* Wrap the tofu in paper towels or a clean dish towel and place it on a plate or cutting board. Put a heavy skillet or pan on top to apply pressure and leave it for at least 30 minutes (longer for a firmer texture). Cut the tofu into 1-inch cubes.
2. In a medium bowl, whisk together 1 tablespoon of oil and the soy sauce and apple cider vinegar. Add the tofu chunks and toss to evenly coat. Cover the bowl and place in the refrigerator to marinate for at least 20 minutes or up to 3 hours.
3. In the meantime, fill three-quarters of a medium saucepan with water and bring to a boil over high heat. Stir in the soba noodles and cook until the noodles are al dente, about 8 minutes. Drain the noodles and transfer to a large bowl to cool for at least 10 minutes.
4. *For the vegetables:* In a medium bowl, whisk together the water, almond butter, lemon juice, and salt.
5. In a large wok, heat 2 tablespoons of the oil over high heat. Once the oil is shimmering, add the carrots, mushrooms, and green onions, and cook until they begin to soften, about 4 minutes. Add the bok choy and cook until wilted, about 5 minutes. Add the almond butter sauce and toss to evenly coat.
6. Transfer the vegetables with the sauce into the bowl with the noodles. Add the cilantro and toss to combine. Clean the wok with a paper towel.

7. In the same wok, heat the remaining 1 tablespoon of oil over high heat. Once the oil is shimmering, add the tofu, shaking off the excess marinade. Cook until browned, about 6 minutes, tossing occasionally. Spoon the tofu over the noodles and sprinkle with the almonds.

8. *To serve*: In each of four bowls, spoon 1⅔ cups of the warm noodle mixture.

9. *To meal prep:* In each of four resealable containers, place 1⅔ cups of the noodle mixture. Cover and refrigerate for up to 4 days or freeze for up to 2 months. To defrost, transfer to the refrigerator for at least 24 hours or up to 4 days.

10. *To reheat*: Transfer the noodles to a microwave-safe bowl and microwave on high for 1½ minutes; let stand for 2 minutes to allow the heat to distribute evenly. Stir and enjoy.

Nutrition Information (per serving): Calories 408; Total Fat 23g; Saturated Fat 3g; Protein 18g; Total Carbohydrates 39g; Fiber 4g; Total Sugars 4g (Includes Added Sugars 0g); Sodium 533mg

Toby's Tip: When reheating, add a few tablespoons of water before microwaving for tender and moist noodles.

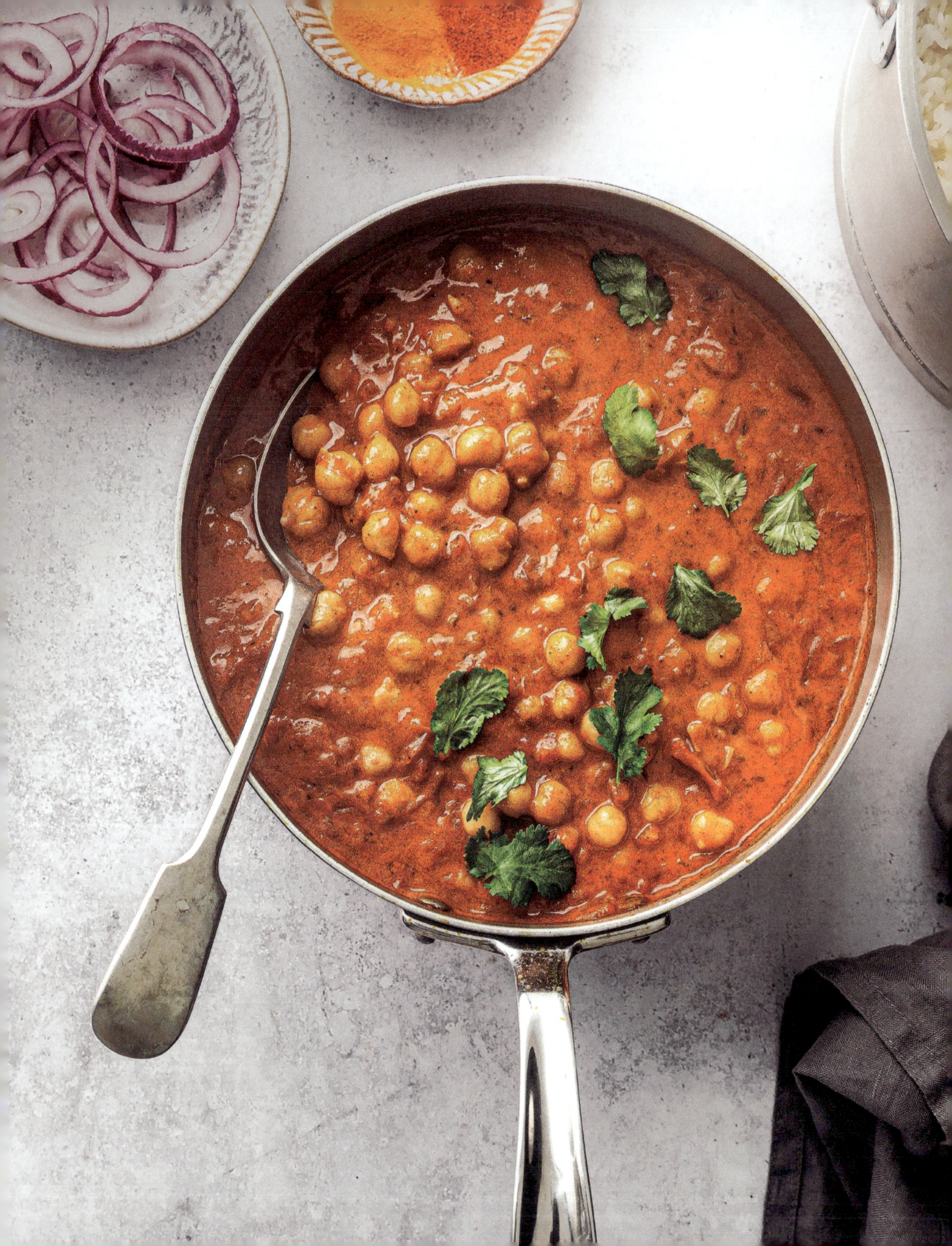

Chickpea Curry

Fuel your body and keep cravings at bay with this satisfying blend. The combination of garbanzo beans and hemp seeds delivers 18 grams of protein and a generous 17 grams of fiber to help you feel fuller for longer.

PREP TIME 20 min // **COOK TIME** 37 min // **TOTAL TIME** 57 min // **SERVINGS** 4 // **SERVING SIZE** 1¼ cups

Meal Prep, Freezer-Friendly, One Pot/Pan | Vegetarian, Dairy-Free

1 tablespoon olive or canola oil
1 medium yellow onion, chopped
1 clove garlic, minced
2 medium carrots, chopped
2 stalks celery, chopped
2 (15.5-ounce) cans low-sodium chickpeas, rinsed and drained
1 (14.5-ounce) can diced tomatoes, with juice
½ cup light coconut milk (45 calories per cup)
½ cup low-sodium vegetable broth
2 tablespoons ground hemp seeds
1 tablespoon reduced-sodium soy sauce
1 teaspoon curry powder
1 teaspoon ground turmeric
¼ teaspoon ground ginger
4 slices whole-grain crusty bread
Optional: chopped cilantro or parsley

1. Heat the oil in a medium pot over medium heat. Once it is shimmering, add the onion and garlic, and cook until fragrant, about 2 minutes. Add the carrots and celery, and cook until softened, about 5 minutes. Stir in the chickpeas, tomatoes, coconut milk, broth, hemp seeds, soy sauce, curry powder, turmeric, and ginger. Increase the heat to high and bring to a boil. Reduce the heat to low, cover, and simmer until the flavors meld, about 30 minutes.
2. *To serve:* In each of four bowls spoon 1¼ cups of the curry and garnish with chopped cilantro or parsley. Serve with 1 slice of bread, for dipping.
3. *To meal prep:* In each of four resealable containers, spoon 1¼ cups of the curry. Refrigerate for up to 4 days or freeze for up to 2 months. To defrost, transfer container to the refrigerator and let thaw for at least 24 hours.
4. *To reheat:* Transfer the curry to a microwave-safe bowl and microwave on high for 1½ minutes; allow to stand for 2 minutes, then stir and serve. Alternatively, place curry in a small saucepan and bring to a boil over high heat. Reduce the heat to medium-low and cook for 10 minutes. Serve warm.

Nutrition Information (per serving): Calories 309; Total Fat 7g; Saturated Fat 1g; Protein 18g; Total Carbohydrates 57g; Fiber 17g; Total Sugars 12g (Includes Added Sugars 0g); Sodium 910mg

Toby's Tip: To balance this dish, serve with the Everyday Side Salad with Red Wine Vinaigrette on page 246.

Cajun-Spiced Red Bean Burgers *with* Scallion Aioli

These plant-forward high-protein burgers offer a bold, smoky, and earthy flavor with a satisfying kick of heat. Served with a cooling and aromatic aioli, they are sure to become a new favorite.

PREP TIME 30 min // **COOK TIME** 10 min // **TOTAL TIME** 40 min // **SERVINGS** 4 // **SERVING SIZE** 1 burger

Meal Prep | **Vegetarian**

FOR THE PATTIES

1 (15.5-ounce) can low-sodium kidney beans, rinsed and drained

1¼ cups rolled oats

1 medium yellow onion, roughly chopped

1 large egg

2 scallions, greens and whites, roughly chopped

2 cloves garlic, crushed

2 tablespoons ground hemp seeds

1½ teaspoons Cajun seasoning

1 teaspoon dried thyme

1 teaspoon sweet paprika

1 teaspoon ground cumin

½ teaspoon kosher salt

Nonstick cooking spray

FOR THE SCALLION AIOLI

1 teaspoon olive, avocado, or canola oil

2 scallions, greens and whites, chopped

¼ cup light mayonnaise

¼ cup plain reduced-fat Greek yogurt

1 clove garlic, minced

1 teaspoon lemon juice

⅛ teaspoon ground paprika

FOR THE BURGER

4 whole-wheat burger buns

4 slices reduced-fat Provolone cheese

8 romaine lettuce leaves

2 plum tomatoes, thinly sliced

1. *For the patties:* In a blender, add the beans, oats, onion, egg, scallions, garlic, hemp seeds, Cajun seasoning, thyme, sweet paprika, cumin, and salt; cover and pulse on high until combined, about 1 minute. Using a spatula, scrape down the sides of the blender, cover, and continue to pulse on high until thoroughly combined, about 1 minute more.

2. Coat a large skillet with cooking spray. Once the oil is shimmering, pour ½ cup of the batter into the pan in a patty shape. Repeat for a second burger, leaving 2 inches between patties. Cook until browned on each side and cooked through, 3 to 4 minutes on each side. Using a spatula, transfer the patties to a clean plate. Repeat with the remaining batter, coating the pan in cooking spray before cooking each set of patties.

3. *For the aioli:* Heat the oil in the same skillet over medium heat. Once the oil is shimmering, add the scallions and sauté until softened, about 2 minutes. Using a spatula, transfer the scallions to a medium bowl and allow to cool for 5 minutes. Add the mayonnaise, yogurt, garlic, lemon juice, and paprika, and whisk to combine.
4. *To serve:* Spread 1 tablespoon of the aioli on each side of 4 buns. Layer with 1 slice of cheese, 2 lettuce leaves, several slices of tomato, and 1 burger. Serve warm.
5. *To meal prep:* Store the burgers, aioli, and buns and vegetables in separate resealable containers in the refrigerator for up to 4 days.
6. *To reheat*: Transfer the burger to a microwave-safe plate and reheat in the microwave for about 1 minute. Allow the heat to evenly distribute for 2 minutes before removing from the microwave and building the burger.

Nutrition Information (per serving): Calories 557; Total Fat 16g; Saturated Fat 4g; Protein 26g; Total Carbohydrates 81g; Fiber 14g; Total Sugars 13g (Includes Added Sugars 0g); Sodium 1,049mg

Toby's Tip: Serve the burger patties over a salad instead of in a bun.

Sheet Pan Eggs *with* Chickpeas and Vegetables

This flavorful sheet-pan dish features a balance of vegetables, beans, and eggs. The secret is za'atar, a Middle Eastern spice blend that gives it a wonderfully tangy and lemony kick.

PREP TIME 25 min // **COOK TIME** 45 min // **TOTAL TIME** 1 hour, 10 min // **SERVINGS** 6

SERVING SIZE 1½ cups

Meal Prep, Freezer-Friendly, One pot/pan | **Vegetarian, Gluten-Free**

Nonstick cooking spray

3 tablespoons extra-virgin olive oil, divided

¾ teaspoon kosher salt, divided

⅜ teaspoon ground black pepper, divided

3 red potatoes, cut into 2-inch cubes

2 teaspoons za'atar seasoning

1 teaspoon ground thyme

⅛ teaspoon red pepper flakes

1 (15.5-ounce) can low-sodium chickpeas, rinsed and drained

1 (10-ounce) container button mushrooms, cut in half

3 plum tomatoes, roughly chopped

1 green bell pepper, seeds and ribs removed, cut into 1-inch strips

1 medium red onion, cut into 1-inch strips

2 cups loosely packed baby spinach

2 tablespoons ground hemp seeds

2 tablespoons raw unsalted sesame seeds

6 large eggs

6 tablespoons full-fat feta cheese, crumbled

3 large whole-wheat pitas, halved

1. Preheat the oven to 400°F. Coat a rimmed baking sheet with nonstick cooking spray.
2. In a large bowl, whisk together 1 tablespoon of the oil, ¼ teaspoon salt, and ⅛ teaspoon black pepper. Add the potatoes and toss to evenly coat. Arrange the potatoes in a single layer on the prepared baking sheet. Place the pan in the preheated oven and roast, turning halfway through, for about 20 minutes.
3. In the same large bowl, add the remaining 2 tablespoons of oil, za'atar, thyme, red pepper flakes, and remaining ½ teaspoon salt and ¼ teaspoon black pepper. Add the chickpeas, mushrooms, tomatoes, pepper, onion, and spinach, and toss to evenly coat in the oil. Carefully transfer the vegetables to the baking sheet with the potatoes and spread evenly. Continue to roast in the oven until the vegetables begin to brown, tossing halfway through, about 15 minutes.
4. Remove the baking sheet from the oven (leave the heat on). Sprinkle the vegetables with the hemp seeds and stir to combine. Sprinkle the sesame seeds overtop.

5. Using the back of a wooden spoon, create 6 wells at least 2 inches apart within the vegetables. Carefully break 1 egg into each of the wells. Place the baking sheet back into the oven and bake until the eggs are cooked through, 8 to 10 minutes.
6. Carefully remove the baking sheet from the oven and sprinkle each egg with 1 tablespoon of the feta cheese.
7. *To serve:* Into each of six bowls spoon 1½ cups of vegetables with 1 egg; serve each with a pita half. Enjoy warm.
8. *To meal prep:* Into each of six resealable containers, spoon 1½ cups of the vegetables with 1 egg. Cover and refrigerate for up to 4 days or freeze for up to 2 months.
9. *To reheat:* To defrost, transfer the container to the refrigerator for 24 hours or up to 4 days. To reheat, transfer the vegetables with egg onto a microwave-safe dish and microwave on high for 1½ minutes; let stand for 2 minutes to allow the heat to distribute evenly. Serve each with half a pita.

Nutrition Information (per serving): Calories 407; Total Fat 16g; Saturated Fat 4g; Protein 20g; Total Carbohydrates 49g; Fiber 10g; Total Sugars 6g (Includes Added Sugars 0g); Sodium 548mg

Toby's Tip: You can find za'atar at your local market in the spice or international aisle, at specialty markets, or online retailers. It complements tofu, eggs, fish, chicken, pork, and lamb beautifully.

Mac and Cheese *with* Edamame and Broccoli

Who doesn't love a cozy bowl of mac and cheese? Take this comfort food to the next level with a delicious plant-based protein twist.

PREP TIME 20 min // **COOK TIME** 20 min // **TOTAL TIME** 40 min // **SERVINGS** 6 // **SERVING SIZE** 1½ cups

Meal Prep, Freezer-Friendly | Vegetarian

Nonstick cooking spray

8 ounces dried elbow macaroni

1½ cups frozen shelled edamame

2 cups broccoli florets, chopped

6 tablespoons unsalted butter, divided

¼ cup all-purpose flour

½ teaspoon mustard powder

½ teaspoon garlic powder

¼ teaspoon kosher salt

⅛ teaspoon cayenne pepper

2 cups reduced-fat ultra-filtered milk (13 grams protein per 1 cup serving), slightly warmed

1½ cups reduced-fat shredded sharp cheddar cheese, divided

¾ cup unseasoned panko breadcrumbs

1. Coat an 8 × 8-inch baking dish with nonstick cooking spray.
2. Fill a medium pot three-quarters with water and bring to a boil. Add the pasta and cook for 2 minutes. Then add the edamame and cook until the pasta is al dente and edamame is cooked through, about 6 minutes more. Transfer to a colander, rinse in cool water, and let drain. Set aside.
3. Fill the same medium pot with 1 inch of water and fit with a steaming basket. Bring to a boil over high heat. Add the broccoli, cover, and cook until the broccoli is just tender, about 5 minutes. Transfer the broccoli to a medium bowl and set aside.
4. In a large saucepan over medium heat, melt 4 tablespoons of the butter. Gradually whisk in the flour, whisking continuously to prevent lumps. Add the mustard, garlic powder, salt, and cayenne, and cook for 1 minute. While whisking, add one-third of the warmed milk and whisk until fully incorporated. Continue whisking in the remaining milk until the mixture is smooth and milk is fully incorporated. Continue cooking for an additional 2 to 3 minutes. Add 1¼ cups of the cheddar cheese and stir until combined and mixture is smooth. Remove the saucepan from the heat. Gently fold in the macaroni mixture and broccoli until combined.
5. Carefully pour the macaroni and cheese mixture into the prepared baking dish.

6. To make the breadcrumbs, melt the remaining 2 tablespoons butter in a small saucepan over low heat. Add the panko breadcrumbs and toss to coat. Toast the breadcrumbs until lightly browned, about 3 minutes. Remove the pan from the heat. Evenly sprinkle the remaining ¼ cup cheddar cheese over the macaroni dish and then sprinkle with the toasted breadcrumbs.
7. *To serve:* On each of six plates, spoon 1½ cups of the macaroni and cheese; enjoy warm.
8. *To meal prep:* In each of six resealable containers, place 1½ cups of the macaroni and cheese. Cover and refrigerate for up to 4 days or freeze for up to 2 months.
9. *To reheat:* To defrost, transfer to the refrigerator for 24 hours. Transfer mac and cheese to a microwave-safe plate and microwave on high for 1½ minutes; let the bowl stand for 2 minutes to allow heat to evenly distribute.

Nutrition Information (per serving): Calories 443; Total Fat 20g; Saturated Fat 13g; Protein 21g; Total Carbohydrates 43g; Fiber 3g; Total Sugars 5g (Includes Added Sugars 0g); Sodium 321mg

Toby's Tip: Swap in cauliflower or carrots for the broccoli.

Quinoa and Kale Bowls *with* Poached Egg

Bowls are more popular than ever because you can easily balance flavors, textures, and nutritious foods for a satisfying, healthy meal. This bowl features protein-filled quinoa with beans and earthy kale mixed with sweet tomatoes —all topped with a delicious poached egg.

PREP TIME 20 min // **COOK TIME** 32 min // **TOTAL TIME** 52 min // **SERVINGS** 4 // **SERVING SIZE** 1 bowl

Meal Prep | **Vegetarian, Gluten-Free, Dairy-Free**

FOR THE QUINOA

1 lemon

1½ cups water

¾ cup dry quinoa

1 teaspoon ground cumin

¼ teaspoon kosher salt

¼ teaspoon ground black pepper

1 cup canned low-sodium Great Northern or cannellini beans

¼ cup fresh flat-leaf parsley leaves, chopped

FOR THE KALE AND TOMATOES

1 tablespoon olive oil

2 cloves garlic, minced

1 shallot, chopped

2 cups cherry tomatoes

4 cups loosely packed kale leaves, chopped

1 teaspoon smoked paprika

1 teaspoon dried oregano

¼ teaspoon kosher salt

⅛ teaspoon ground black pepper

FOR THE POACHED EGGS

2 teaspoons unseasoned rice vinegar

4 large eggs

¼ cup chopped walnuts

1. Cut 4 (1-inch) peels from the lemon. Quarter the lemon.
2. *For the quinoa:* In a medium saucepan, stir together the water, quinoa, lemon peel, cumin, salt, and pepper. Bring to a boil over high heat. Reduce the heat to medium-low and simmer, covered, until the quinoa is tender, about 15 minutes. Stir in the beans and parsley, and heat through for an additional 1 to 2 minutes. Fluff with a fork and discard the lemon peel.
3. *For the kale and tomatoes:* Heat the oil in a medium skillet over medium heat. Once the oil is shimmering, add the garlic and shallot and cook until fragrant, about 2 minutes. Add the cherry tomatoes and cook until slightly softened, about 3 minutes. Add the kale and cook until wilted, about 4 minutes. Add the paprika, oregano, salt, and pepper, and toss to evenly coat. Set aside to slightly cool for 5 minutes.

4. *For the eggs:* Fill a medium saucepan three-quarters with water and bring to a boil over high heat. Add the vinegar and reduce the heat until it is no longer at a rolling boil. Crack an egg into a small cup, bowl, or wineglass. Holding it near the surface of the water, gently slide the egg into the gently simmering hot water. Repeat with the remaining eggs. Cover the saucepan and allow the eggs to cook for exactly 6 minutes. Using a slotted spoon, carefully transfer each egg to a paper towel to drain.

5. *To serve*: On one side of each of four bowls, spoon ¾ cup of the quinoa. Spoon 1 cup of the kale mixture onto the other half of the bowl. Top with 1 poached egg. Sprinkle with 1 tablespoon walnuts and place a lemon wedge on the side. Serve warm.

6. *To meal prep*: In each of four containers, prep the quinoa, kale, and egg as above. Cover and refrigerate for up to 4 days.

7. *To reheat*: Remove the lemon wedge and transfer remaining contents into a microwave-safe bowl. Microwave on high for 1½ minutes; let stand for 2 minutes to allow the heat to evenly distribute. Squeeze lemon juice over top before eating.

Nutrition Information (per serving): Calories 405; Total Fat 16g; Saturated Fat 3g; Protein 21g; Total Carbohydrates 48g; Fiber 9g; Total Sugars 4g (Includes Added Sugars 0g); Sodium 402mg

Toby's Tip: Swap the quinoa for amaranth, a whole grain with a similar amount of protein per serving.

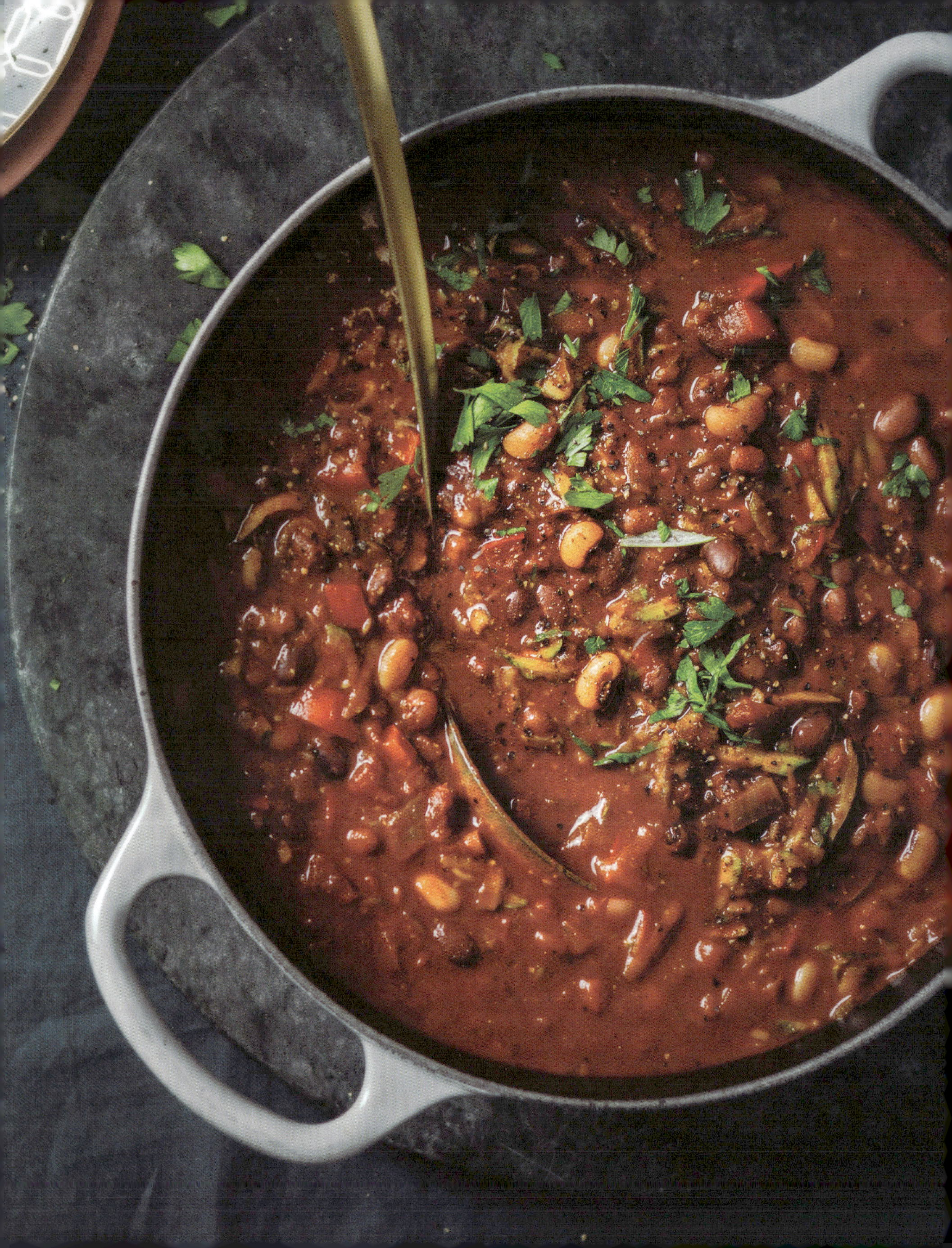

Three-Bean Plant-Forward Chili

Beans pack a powerful protein punch, but did you know that research published by the journal *Maturitas* has shown that eating about 2 servings of beans a day can improve your overall diet quality by 25 percent compared to people who don't eat beans? Plus, beans provide fiber and potassium, nutrients that most people fall short on.

PREP TIME 20 min // **COOK TIME** 38 min // **TOTAL TIME** 58 min // **SERVINGS** 6 // **SERVING SIZE** 1⅓ cups

Meal Prep, Freezer-Friendly, One Pot/Pan | Vegetarian

2 tablespoons olive oil

1 medium onion, chopped

2 cloves garlic, minced

1 jalapeño pepper, seeds and ribs removed, roughly chopped

2 stalks celery, roughly chopped

2 medium carrots, roughly chopped

1 (15.5-ounce) can low-sodium kidney beans, rinsed and drained

1 (15-ounce) can low-sodium pinto beans, rinsed and drained

1 (15.5-ounce) can low-sodium black beans, rinsed and drained

1 (14.5-ounce) can low-sodium fire-roasted diced tomatoes, with liquid

1½ cups low-sodium vegetable broth

1 (6-ounce) can tomato paste

¼ cup dry quinoa

2 tablespoons ground hemp seeds

1 tablespoon chili powder

2 teaspoons ground oregano

1 teaspoon ground cumin

1 teaspoon liquid honey

½ teaspoon kosher salt

¼ teaspoon cayenne pepper

1 cup plain reduced-fat (2 percent) Greek yogurt

1 cup reduced-fat shredded Mexican cheese blend

1. Heat the oil in a medium pot over medium heat. Once the oil is shimmering, add the onion, garlic, and jalapeño, and cook until the onion is translucent and the garlic is fragrant, about 3 minutes. Add the celery and carrots, and cook until the vegetables soften, about 5 minutes.

2. Add the beans, diced tomatoes, broth, tomato paste, quinoa, hemp seeds, chili powder, oregano, cumin, honey, salt, and cayenne and stir to combine. Increase the heat to high and bring the mixture to a boil. Then reduce the heat to medium -low and simmer, covered, until the flavors meld, about 30 minutes. Stir occasionally during cooking time. Remove the chili from the heat and allow to cool for 10 minutes.

3. *To serve:* In each of six bowls, spoon 1⅓ cups of the chili and top with ¼ cup each of yogurt and cheese. Serve warm.

recipe continues →

4. *To meal prep:* In each of six resealable containers, place 1⅓ cups of the chili and store ¼ cup each of the yogurt and cheese in separate smaller containers. Cover and refrigerate for up to 4 days or freeze for up to 2 months.
5. *To reheat:* To defrost, transfer the frozen container(s) of chili to the refrigerator for 24 hours. Transfer the chili to a microwave-safe bowl and microwave on high for 1½ minutes; let the bowl stand for 2 minutes to allow heat to distribute evenly.

Nutrition Information (per serving): Calories 414; Total Fat 11g; Saturated Fat 3g; Protein 25g; Total Carbohydrates 57g; Fiber 19g; Total Sugars 12g (Includes Added Sugars 1g); Sodium 863mg

Toby's Tip: There are several types of oils you can use on the stove top instead of olive oil, including canola, sunflower, and avocado oil.

Broccoli, Cauliflower, and Farro Casserole

Cottage cheese is the secret to this creamy, high-protein casserole. It adds a custardy texture and a hint of tang, with roughly 13 grams of protein in every half-cup.

PREP TIME 20 min // **COOK TIME** 54 min // **TOTAL TIME** 1 hour, 14 min // **SERVINGS** 6 // **SERVING SIZE** 1⅓ cups

Meal Prep, Freezer-Friendly | **Vegetarian**

- 1 cup dry farro
- 3 cups low-sodium vegetable broth or water
- Nonstick cooking spray
- 1 tablespoon olive oil
- 1 medium yellow onion, chopped
- 2 cloves garlic, minced
- 2 cups bite-size broccoli florets
- 2 cups bite-size cauliflower florets
- 1 cup cherry tomatoes
- 1 cup low-fat (1 percent) cottage cheese
- 1¼ cups reduced-fat shredded cheddar cheese
- 2 large eggs, beaten
- 1 teaspoon Dijon mustard
- ½ teaspoon ground paprika
- ¼ teaspoon kosher salt
- ¼ teaspoon ground black pepper
- ½ cup unseasoned panko breadcrumbs

1. In a medium saucepan, add the farro and broth or water and bring to a boil over high heat. Reduce the heat to medium-low, cover, and simmer until fluffy, 25 to 30 minutes. Fluff the farro with a fork, remove the pan from the heat, and allow to slightly cool for 10 minutes.
2. Preheat the oven to 375°F. Coat an 8 × 11.5-inch baking dish with cooking spray.
3. Heat the oil in a medium skillet over medium heat. Once the oil is shimmering, add the onion and garlic, and cook until the onion is softened and garlic is fragrant, about 2 minutes. Add the broccoli, cauliflower, and tomatoes, and toss to combine. Cook until the vegetables are slightly softened, 6 to 7 minutes. Remove the pan from the heat and allow to slightly cool for 10 minutes.
4. In a large bowl, mix together the cottage cheese, cheddar cheese, eggs, mustard, paprika, salt, and pepper. Add the farro and vegetables, and toss to evenly coat. Transfer the mixture to the prepared baking dish, spreading into an even layer. Sprinkle with the breadcrumbs.
5. Cover the baking dish with aluminum foil and transfer to the preheated oven. Cook for 15 minutes and then uncover and continue baking until the breadcrumbs are slightly browned, an additional 15 minutes. Remove the casserole from the oven and allow to set for 15 minutes.
6. *To serve:* Into each of six bowls, spoon 1⅓ cups of the casserole; serve warm.

recipe continues 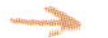

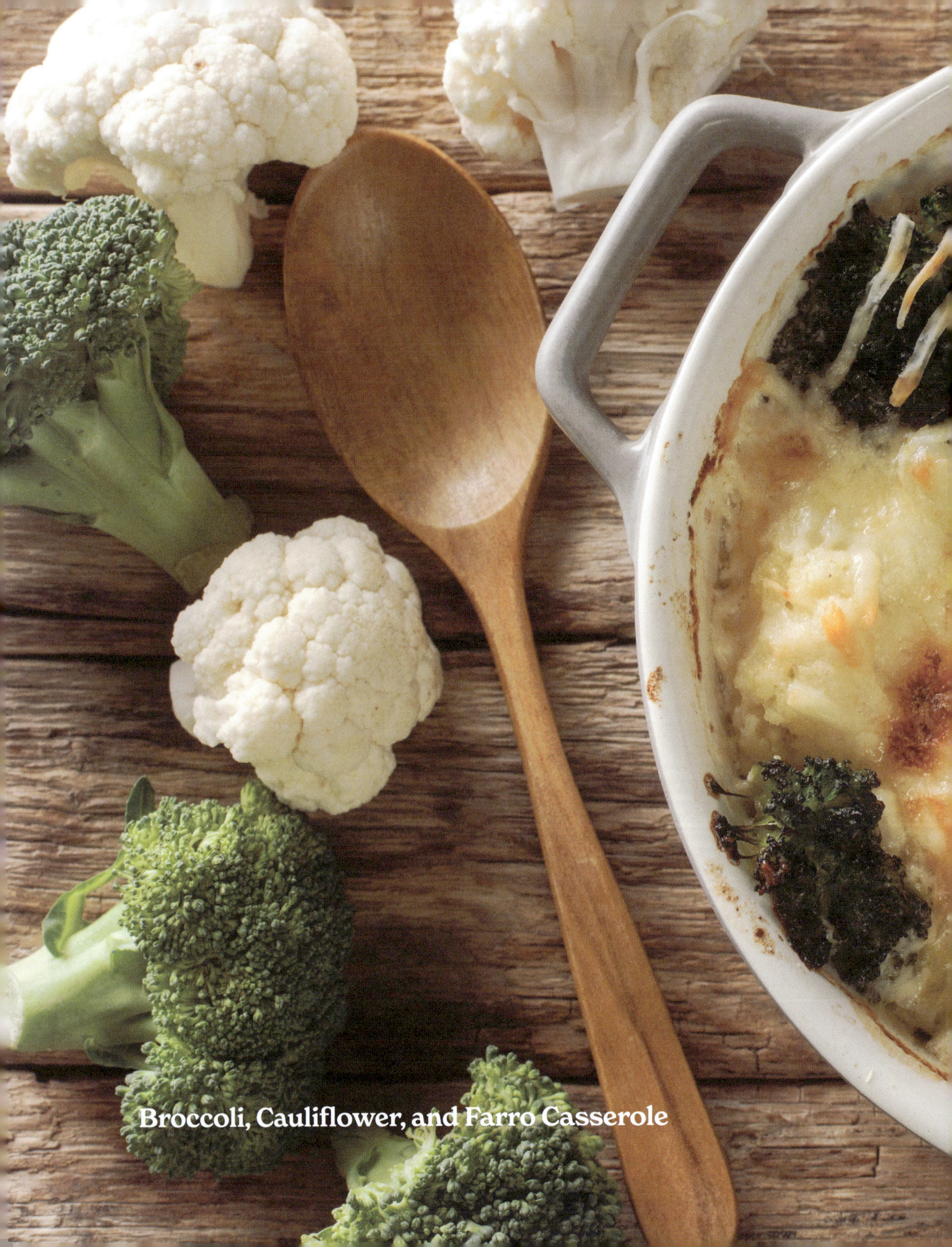

Broccoli, Cauliflower, and Farro Casserole

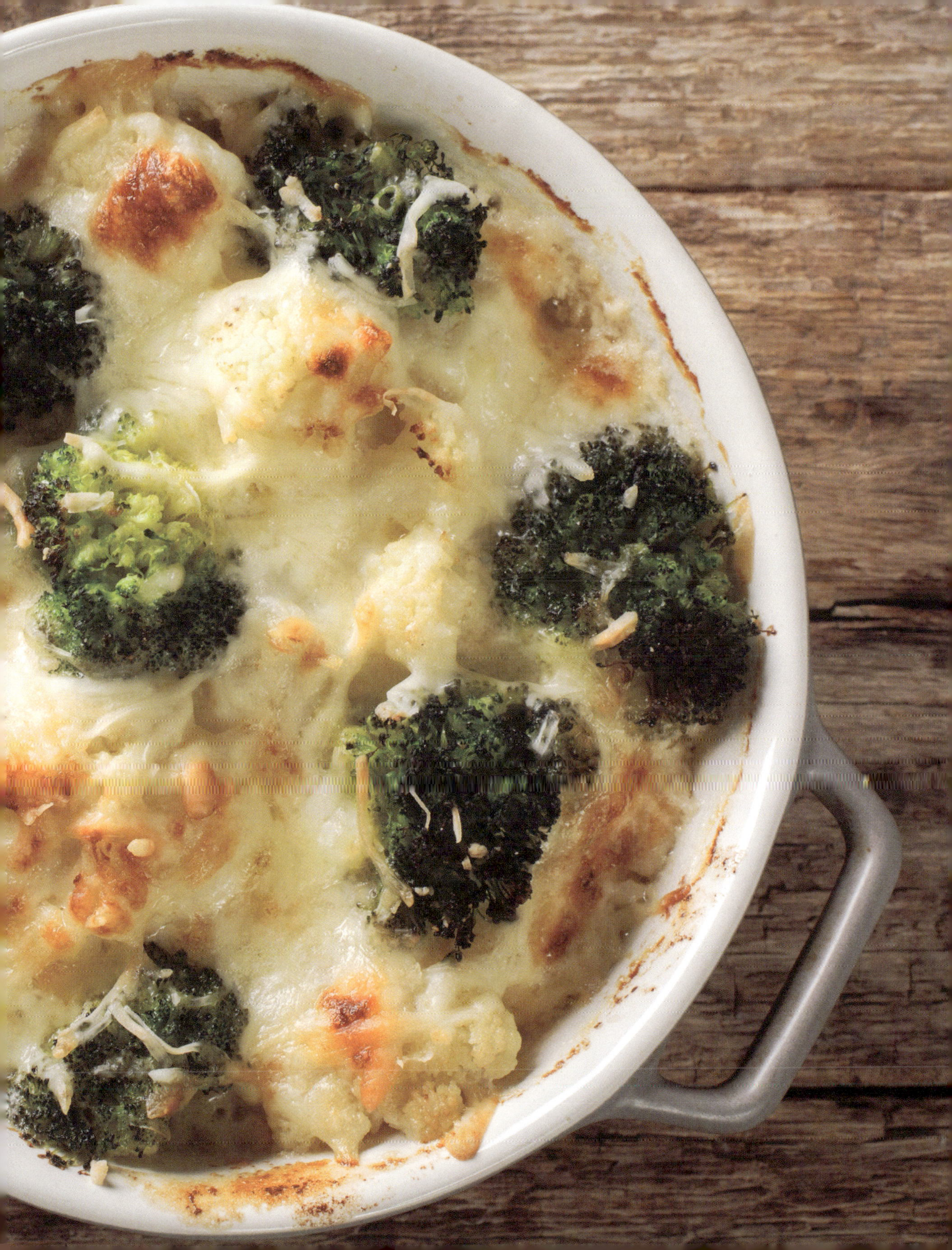

7. *To meal prep:* In each of six resealable containers, spoon 1⅓ cups of the casserole. Cover and refrigerate for up to 4 days or freeze for up to 2 months.

8. *To reheat:* To defrost, transfer to the refrigerator for 24 hours or up to 4 days. To reheat, transfer the casserole to a microwave-safe bowl and microwave on high for 1½ minutes; let stand for 2 minutes to allow the heat to evenly distribute.

Nutrition Information (per serving): Calories 304; Total Fat 10g; Saturated Fat 4g; Protein 20g; Total Carbohydrates 34g; Fiber 6g; Total Sugars 4g (Includes Added Sugars 0g); Sodium 508mg

Toby's Tip: Swap brown rice for farro, which has a similar amount of protein per serving.

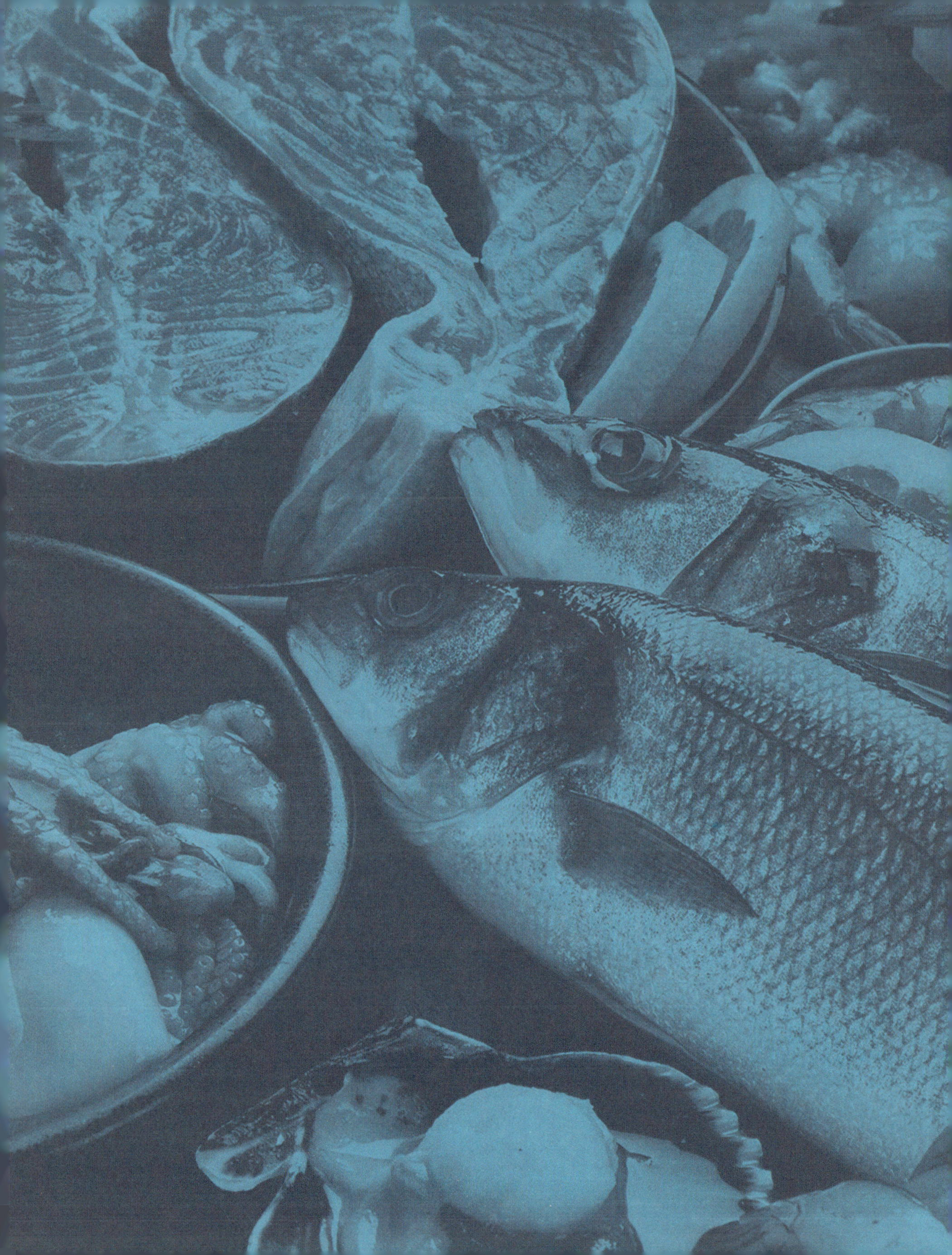

CHAPTER 8

Fish and Seafood Mains

Crab Cake Bowls *with* Brown Rice and Swiss Chard

Satisfy your appetite with this 27-gram protein bowl, featuring zesty Old Bay crab cakes, Swiss chard, and rice.

PREP TIME 40 min // **COOK TIME** 1 hour, 5 min // **TOTAL TIME** 1 hour, 45 min

SERVINGS 4 // **SERVING SIZE** 1 bowl

Meal Prep | **Vegetarian**

FOR THE BROWN RICE

1 tablespoon olive oil

3 scallions, greens and whites, chopped

⅔ cup dry brown rice

2 cups water

1 cup frozen peas and carrots

¼ teaspoon kosher salt

⅛ teaspoon ground black pepper

3 tablespoons fresh flat-leaf parsley leaves, chopped

FOR THE SWISS CHARD

1 bunch rainbow or Swiss chard, thick stems trimmed

1 tablespoon olive oil

1 medium yellow onion, cut into ¾-inch pieces

2 cloves garlic, minced

1 cup low-sodium chickpeas, rinsed and drained

1 tablespoon lemon juice

¼ teaspoon kosher salt

FOR THE CRAB CAKES

1 large egg

1 scallion, greens and whites, roughly chopped

1 clove garlic, crushed

1 tablespoon lemon juice

1 teaspoon Dijon mustard

1 teaspoon Old Bay seasoning

1 teaspoon Worcestershire sauce

1 pound lump crab meat

¾ cup unseasoned panko breadcrumbs

2 tablespoons olive or canola oil

1. *For the brown rice:* Heat the oil in a medium saucepan over medium heat. Once the oil is shimmering, add the scallions and cook until fragrant, about 2 minutes. Add the rice, water, peas and carrots, salt, and pepper, and bring to a boil over high heat. Reduce the heat to low and simmer, covered, until the rice is tender and water is absorbed, 40 minutes. Add parsley and toss to combine; keep warm.
2. *For the Swiss chard:* Roughly slice each leaf with the stem into thirds.

3. Heat the oil in a large skillet over medium heat. Once the oil is shimmering, add the onion and garlic, and cook until the onion has softened and the garlic is fragrant, about 3 minutes. Add the Swiss chard and cook until wilted, about 4 minutes. Turn off the heat and stir in the chickpeas, lemon juice, and salt; toss to combine.

4. *For the crab cakes:* In a medium bowl, whisk together the egg, scallion, garlic, lemon juice, mustard, Old Bay seasoning, and Worcestershire sauce. Add the crab meat and panko and toss gently to combine. Transfer the mixture to a blender or food processor, and pulse about 10 times for 5 seconds each time, until the crab meat is well combined.

5. Scoop out 1 tablespoon of the crab mixture and, using clean hands, form into a patty. Place on a large plate and gently press down with the palm of your hand to flatten slightly. Repeat to make 12 crab cakes. Cover with plastic wrap and refrigerate for at least 20 minutes or up to 1 hour.

6. In a large pan, heat the oil over medium heat. Once the oil is shimmering, add 6 crab cakes, spacing each about 1 inch apart. Sauté until golden brown, about 4 minutes on one side. Then flip and cook, covered, for 2 minutes. Remove the cover and cook for 2 minutes more. Transfer the cooked crab cakes to a plate, cover with foil to keep warm, and repeat with the remaining crab cakes.

7. *To serve:* In each of four bowls, spoon ¾ cup rice and 1 cup chard, and top with 3 crab cakes. Serve warm.

8. *To meal prep:* Prepare the rice, chard, and crab cakes as above in four resealable containers. Cover and refrigerate for up to 4 days.

9. *To reheat*: Transfer to a microwave-safe plate and microwave on high for 1 minute; let stand for 2 minutes to allow the heat to distribute evenly.

Nutrition Information (per serving): Calories 450; Total Fat 19g; Saturated Fat 3g; Protein 27g; Total Carbohydrates 46g; Fiber 8g; Total Sugars 7g (Includes Added Sugars 0g); Sodium 1,314mg

Toby's Tip: Swap the Swiss chard for kale, spinach, collard greens, or beet greens.

Sesame-Crusted Seared Tuna Poke Bowls

My Gen Z daughters are constantly recreating poke bowls they see on social media. When I whipped these up, my daughters stopped recreating what they saw online and made these their go-to poke bowls.

PREP TIME 20 min // **COOK TIME** 25 min // **TOTAL TIME** 45 min // **SERVINGS** 4 // **SERVING SIZE** 1 bowl

Vegetarian, Dairy-Free

FOR THE RICE

1 cup dry sushi rice

2 cups water

2 tablespoons unseasoned rice vinegar

2 teaspoon liquid honey

½ teaspoon kosher salt

FOR THE TUNA

1 tablespoon reduced-sodium soy sauce

1 tablespoon liquid honey

1½ pounds ahi tuna

3 tablespoons raw sesame seeds

1 teaspoon ground thyme

¼ teaspoon onion powder

¼ teaspoon kosher salt

⅛ teaspoon ground black pepper

2 tablespoons olive oil

1 cup frozen shelled edamame

FOR THE SOY DRESSING

¼ cup reduced-sodium soy sauce

1 teaspoon sesame oil

1 teaspoon liquid honey

2 Persian or Kirby (mini) cucumbers, cut into 1-inch cubes

2 medium carrots, grated

2 medium scallions, greens and whites, chopped

1 (0.35-ounce) package of sea salt seaweed snacks

1. *For the rice:* Place the rice and water in a medium saucepan and bring to a boil over high heat. Reduce the heat to medium-low, cover, and simmer until tender, about 15 minutes. Transfer to a medium bowl and fluff with a fork.
2. In a small bowl, whisk together the rice vinegar, honey, and salt. Pour it over the cooked rice and toss to evenly coat.
3. *For the tuna:* In a small bowl, whisk together the soy sauce and honey. Brush the soy-honey mixture over both sides of the tuna and place the tuna on a large plate.
4. In another small bowl, stir together the sesame seeds, thyme, onion powder, salt, and pepper. Sprinkle one side of the tuna with half the sesame seed mixture and press it down with clean hands; repeat on the opposite side.

5. Heat the oil in a large saucepan over medium-high heat. Once the oil is shimmering and very hot, place the tuna into the pan, gently pressing it down with a spatula. Cook until the bottom is browned, about 1½ minutes, and then flip over and brown the other side, another 1½ minutes. Using tongs, carefully stand up the tuna and cook the edges about 1 minute. Transfer the tuna to a cutting board and allow to cool for 10 minutes. Using a sharp knife, thinly slice the tuna about 1 inch thick and set aside.
6. *For the toppings:* Fill a small saucepan three-quarters with water and bring to a boil over high heat. Add the edamame and then reduce the heat to medium-low. Cook until the edamame is tender, about 5 minutes. Drain and allow the edamame to slightly cool for 10 minutes.
7. *For the soy dressing:* In a small bowl, whisk together the soy sauce, sesame oil, and honey.
8. *To serve:* In each of four bowls, spoon ¾ cup of rice. On one side of the bowl, top the rice with one-quarter of the tuna. Next, top the other side of the bowl with ¼ cup of edamame and one-quarter of the cucumbers, carrots, and scallions. Drizzle with 1 tablespoon of the dressing. Serve with one-quarter of the seaweed pieces for scooping.

Nutrition Information (per serving): Calories 614; Total Fat 22g; Saturated Fat 4g; Protein 50g; Total Carbohydrates 55g; Fiber 5g; Total Sugars 12g (Includes Added Sugars 8g); Sodium 744mg

Toby's Tip: Use the seaweed snack pieces to scoop the poke or sub in seaweed salad and use it as a topping.

Sardines in Tomato Sauce over Couscous

Sardines provide not only protein but also a hefty dose of omega-3 fats. The American Heart Association recommends eating two servings (3 to 4 ounces cooked) of fish per week (especially fatty fish like sardines, tuna, and salmon) as part of a heart-healthy diet.

PREP TIME 20 min // **COOK TIME** 20 min // **TOTAL TIME** 40 min // **SERVINGS** 4

SERVING SIZE 1⅓ cups + ¾ cup couscous

Meal Prep, Freezer-Friendly, One Pot/Pan | Vegetarian, Dairy-Free

- 1 tablespoon olive oil
- 1 medium yellow onion, cut into ¾-inch strips
- 2 cloves garlic, minced
- 2 green bell peppers, seeds and ribs removed, cut into ¾-inch strips
- 1 (10-ounce) container cremini mushrooms, thinly sliced
- 1 (28-ounce) can crushed tomatoes
- ¼ cup low-sodium vegetable broth or water
- 2 (3.75-ounce) cans sardines in water, drained
- 1 teaspoon ground paprika
- 1 teaspoon ground cumin
- 1 teaspoon dried oregano
- ½ teaspoon kosher salt
- ¼ teaspoon ground black pepper
- 1½ cups water
- 1 cup dry pearled couscous

1. Heat the oil in a large skillet over medium heat. Once the oil is shimmering, add the onion and garlic, and cook until the onion is translucent and garlic is fragrant, about 3 minutes. Add the peppers and mushrooms, and cook until the vegetables begin to soften, about 5 minutes. Add the crushed tomatoes, broth or water, sardines, paprika, cumin, oregano, salt, and black pepper, and stir to combine. Bring the mixture to a boil over high heat, then reduce the heat to medium-low and simmer, covered, until the flavors meld, 20 minutes.
2. Bring the water and couscous to a boil in a medium saucepan over high heat. Cover, reduce the heat to medium-low, and simmer until the couscous is tender, about 15 minutes.
3. *To serve:* On each of four plates, spoon about ¾ cup of the couscous and top with 1⅓ cups of the sardines in tomato sauce. Serve warm.
4. *To meal prep:* In each of four resealable containers, spoon ¾ cup of the couscous and top with 1⅓ cups of the sardines in tomato sauce. Cover and refrigerate for up to 4 days or freeze for up to 2 months.

5. *To reheat:* To defrost, transfer to the refrigerator for 24 hours to up to 4 days. To reheat, transfer to a microwave-safe plate and microwave on high for 1½ minutes; let stand for 2 minutes to allow the heat to distribute evenly.

Nutrition Information (per serving): Calories 422; Total Fat 12g; Saturated Fat 2g; Protein 27g; Total Carbohydrates 57g; Fiber 8g; Total Sugars 13g (Includes Added Sugars 0g); Sodium 603mg

Toby's Tip: To make the dish gluten-free, serve over quinoa, rice, or with a gluten-free slice of bread.

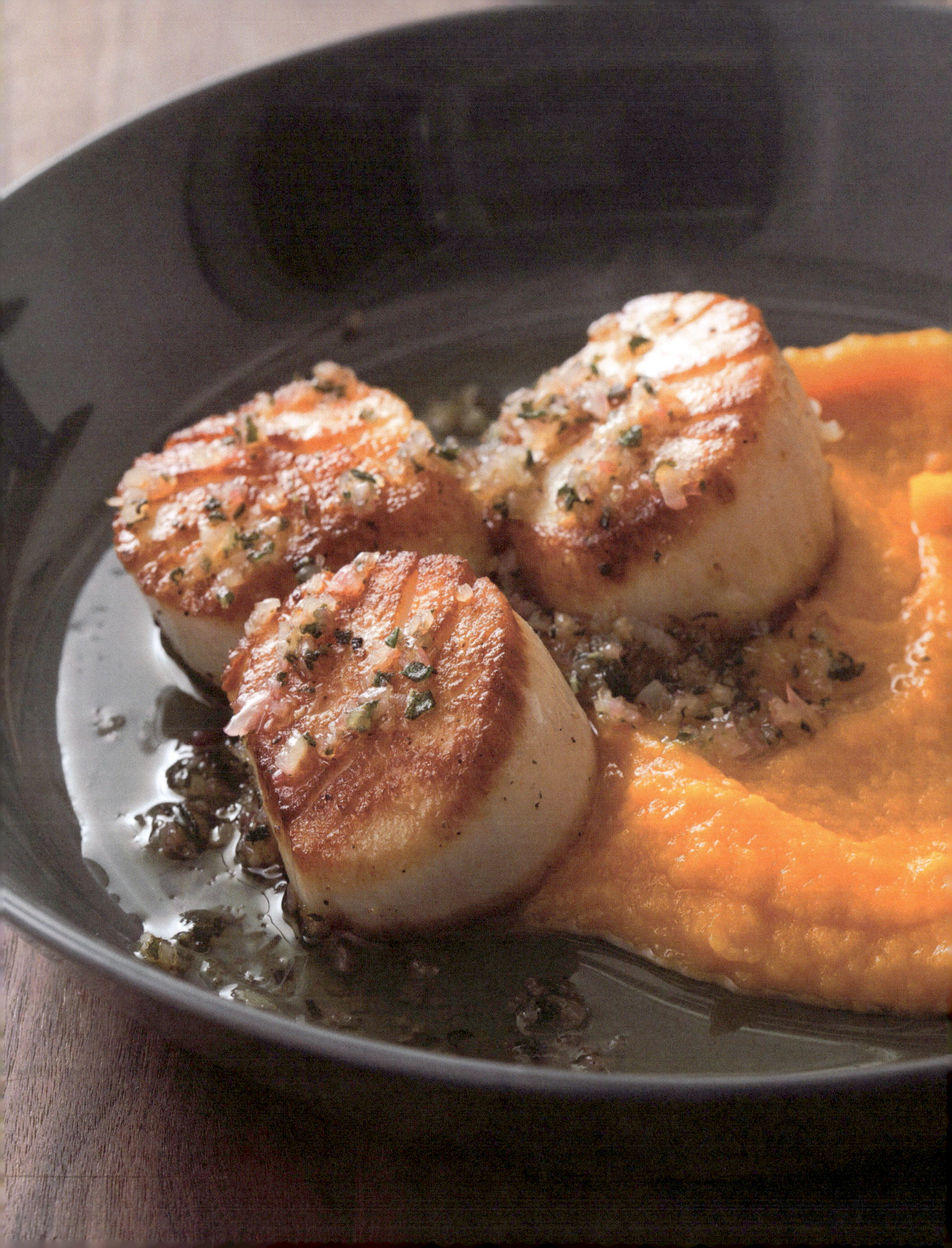

Pan-Fried Scallops with Butternut Squash Purée

This elegant but approachable dish pairs tender, pan-seared scallops with a smooth butternut squash purée for a balanced, protein-forward meal.

PREP TIME 10 min // **COOK TIME** 55 min // **TOTAL TIME** 1 hour, 5 min // **SERVINGS** 4

SERVING SIZE 4 scallops + 1 cup purée

Meal Prep | **Gluten-Free**

FOR THE BUTTERNUT SQUASH

1 large butternut squash, peeled, seeded, and cut in 1-inch cubes

2 tablespoons extra-virgin olive oil

Kosher salt, to taste

Freshly ground black pepper, to taste

1 tablespoon butter

1 small onion, diced

3 garlic cloves

1½ cups vegetable stock

FOR THE SEARED SCALLOPS

16 large sea scallops

3 tablespoons extra-virgin olive oil

1 large shallot, minced

2 garlic cloves, minced

1 tablespoon dried parsley

Kosher salt, to taste

Freshly ground black pepper, to taste

Nutrition Information (per serving): Calories 445; Total Fat 21g; Saturated Fat 5g; Protein 28g; Total Carbohydrates 30g; Dietary Fiber 4g; Total Sugars 6g (Includes Added Sugars 0g); Sodium 720mg

1. *To make the butternut squash:* Preheat the oven to 400°F. In a bowl, toss the squash with the olive oil and season with salt and pepper. Arrange in a single layer on a baking sheet and roast for 35 to 45 minutes, until tender.
2. Melt the butter in a sauté pan over medium heat. Add the onion and garlic and cook until softened, about 5 minutes. Transfer the roasted squash, onion, and garlic to a food processor or blender. Add about 1 cup of the stock and purée until smooth. Add more stock as needed. Season with salt and pepper.
3. *To make the scallops:* Rinse the scallops and pat dry with paper towels. Set aside.
4. Heat the olive oil in a large skillet over medium-high heat. Add the shallot, garlic, and parsley and sauté until softened, about 2 to 3 minutes. Add the scallops and sear until just opaque, about 3 minutes per side.
5. *To serve:* Spoon the purée onto plates. Top with one-quarter of the scallops and drizzle with the pan drippings. Repeat with the remaining ingredients.
6. *To meal prep:* Prepare the butternut squash purée up to 4 days in advance and store in an airtight container in the refrigerator. Reheat gently on the stovetop before serving. Cook the scallops just before eating for best texture and flavor.

Pan-Seared Branzino *with* Parsley Sauce

One of my favorite fish is branzino, which I request filleted from my fishmonger. This version is jazzed up with a refreshing parsley sauce that takes just 5 minutes to whip up.

PREP TIME 20 min // **COOK TIME** 16 min // **TOTAL TIME** 36 min // **SERVINGS** 4

SERVING SIZE 1 fillet + about 2 tablespoons sauce

Meal Prep | **Vegetarian, Gluten-Free**

FOR THE PARSLEY SAUCE

1 cup loosely packed fresh flat-leaf parsley leaves and stems, roughly chopped

1 shallot

1 tablespoon lemon juice

1 clove garlic, smashed

½ teaspoon dried oregano

¼ teaspoon ground cumin

¼ teaspoon kosher salt

½ cup extra-virgin olive oil

FOR THE BRANZINO

4 (4-ounce) branzino fillets

¼ teaspoon kosher salt

¼ teaspoon ground black pepper

2 tablespoons unsalted butter, divided

1. *For the parsley sauce:* In a food processor or blender, combine the parsley, shallot, lemon juice, garlic, oregano, cumin, and salt. Add the oil and pulse until coarsely puréed. Let sit for 1 to 2 minutes to allow the flavors to meld.
2. *For the branzino*: Sprinkle the branzino fillets with the salt and pepper.
3. Heat 1 tablespoon of the butter in a large skillet over medium-high heat. Once the butter is shimmering, add two of the branzino fillets skin-side down and cook until they reach an internal temperature of 145°F, about 4 minutes on each side. Transfer the branzino to a plate and cover with aluminum foil to keep warm. Repeat with the remaining 1 tablespoon of butter and 2 branzino fillets.
4. *To serve:* On each of four plates, place 1 branzino fillet and top with about 2 tablespoons of the parsley sauce. Serve warm.
5. *To meal prep:* In each of four resealable containers, place 1 branzino fillet. In separate small resealable containers, spoon about 2 tablespoons of the sauce. Cover both containers and refrigerate for up to 4 days.

6. *To reheat:* To reheat, transfer onto a microwave-safe plate and microwave on high for 1 minute; allow to sit for 2 minutes for the heat to distribute evenly. Top with parsley sauce and serve.

Nutrition Information (per serving): Calories 413; Total Fat 36g; Saturated Fat 9g; Protein 22g; Total Carbohydrates 3g; Fiber 1g; Total Sugars 1g (Includes Added Sugars 0g); Sodium 242mg

Toby's Tip: Enjoy the parsley sauce over tofu, haddock, cod, chicken, or turkey.

Haddock in Foil *with* Zucchini, Squash, and Red Pepper

What's better than a meal that doesn't need much cleanup? There's no pot or plate needed in this dish—enjoy eating right from the pouch! Just let it cool a few minutes before serving.

PREP TIME 15 min // **COOK TIME** 15 min // **TOTAL TIME** 30 min // **SERVINGS** 4 // **SERVING SIZE** 1 pouch

Meal Prep, One Pot/Pan, 30 Minutes or Less | Vegetarian, Gluten-Free, Dairy-Free

4 (6-ounce) haddock fillets

½ teaspoon kosher salt, divided

½ teaspoon ground black pepper, divided

1 medium zucchini, cut into ½-inch rounds

1 medium yellow squash, cut into ½-inch rounds

1 medium red bell pepper, seeds and ribs removed, cut into ½-inch strips

1 small yellow onion, cut into ½-inch slices

2 lemons, 1 thinly sliced and 1 juiced

2 tablespoons extra-virgin olive oil

2 tablespoons white cooking wine or dry white wine

⅛ teaspoon red pepper flakes

8 basil leaves

1. Preheat the oven to 425°F. Prepare 4 large pieces of aluminum foil or parchment paper. Set aside 2 baking sheets.
2. Sprinkle both sides of the haddock with ¼ teaspoon each of salt and black pepper and position one in the center of each piece of foil or parchment paper. Top each piece of fish with an even amount of zucchini, squash, red pepper, and onion pieces.
3. In a small bowl, whisk together the lemon juice, oil, wine, red pepper flakes, and remaining ¼ teaspoon each salt and pepper. Spoon the lemon juice mixture evenly over each of the fillets, and top with an even amount of basil leaves. Finish each with 2 to 3 lemon slices.
4. Seal the foil or parchment paper, being careful to seal the ends.
5. To cook, place 2 packets on each baking sheet and roast in the preheated oven until the fish is opaque and reaches and internal temperature of 145°F, about 15 minutes. Using a sharp knife, carefully cut several 3-inch slits into the package to allow the steam to release. Allow to stand for about 10 minutes before serving.
6. *To meal prep:* Place cooked fish with contents into each of four resealable containers. Cover and refrigerate for up to 2 days.

7. *To reheat*: Transfer fish with contents onto a microwave-safe plate and microwave on high for 1 minute; let stand for 2 minutes to allow heat to distribute evenly.

Nutrition Information (per serving): Calories 228; Total Fat 8g; Saturated Fat 1g; Protein 30g; Total Carbohydrates 8g; Fiber 2g; Total Sugars 4g (Includes Added Sugars 0g); Sodium 524mg

Toby's Tip: The cooking method used in this recipe is called *en papillote*, where you put food into a folded pouch and then bake it. You can purchase parchment cooking bags or use parchment paper or aluminum foil to create a bag.

Cod Fish Tacos *with* Cabbage Slaw

Taco Tuesday was a beloved ritual when my kids were growing up. Now that they're in college and beyond, the tradition lives on—but tacos have become a meal for any night of the week.

PREP TIME 45 min // **COOK TIME** 10 min // **TOTAL TIME** 55 min // **SERVINGS** 4 // **SERVING SIZE** 2 tacos

Vegetarian, Dairy-Free

FOR THE FISH

⅓ cup + 1 tablespoon extra-virgin olive oil or olive oil

Zest and juice of 1 lime

2 cloves garlic, minced

1 tablespoon liquid honey

1 teaspoon smoked paprika

1 teaspoon chili powder

1 teaspoon ground cumin

½ teaspoon ground oregano

¼ teaspoon kosher salt

¼ teaspoon ground black pepper

1 pound cod fillets

FOR THE SLAW

2 medium carrots, shredded

4 cups loosely packed green cabbage, shredded

¼ cup fresh cilantro leaves and stems, chopped

FOR THE TACOS

Nonstick cooking spray

8 (6-inch) corn tortillas

1 lime, quartered

1. *For the fish:* In a small bowl, whisk together ⅓ cup of the oil, lime zest and juice, garlic, honey, paprika, chili, cumin, oregano, salt, and pepper. Spoon 3 tablespoons of the dressing into a bowl and set aside.
2. Place the fish into a large bowl and toss with the remaining dressing. Cover and refrigerate for 20 minutes or up to 2 hours.
3. Heat the remaining 1 tablespoon of oil in a large skillet over medium heat. Once the oil is shimmering, add the cod, shaking off excess dressing, and cook until it reaches a minimum internal temperature of 145°F, 4 to 5 minutes per side. Transfer the fish to a cutting board and allow to stand for 5 minutes. Using a fork, separate the fish into 2-inch pieces.
4. *For the slaw:* In a large mixing bowl, toss together the carrots, cabbage, and cilantro. Add the 3 tablespoons of the dressing and toss to combine.

5. *For the tacos:* Coat a large skillet with cooking spray and heat over medium-low heat. Place 1 tortilla in the skillet and heat for 1 minute on each side, until warmed through. Transfer to a plate and cover with a clean cloth or paper towel. Repeat for the remaining tortillas.

6. *To serve:* On each of four plates, place 2 tortillas. In each tortilla, spoon 2 tablespoons of the slaw and top with an even amount of the cod strips. Place a lime quarter onto each piece and serve.

Nutrition Information (per serving): Calories 511; Total Fat 34g; Saturated Fat 5g; Protein 25g; Total Carbohydrates 32g; Fiber 7g; Total Sugars 5g (Includes Added Sugars 0g); Sodium 199mg

Toby's Tip: Swap the cod for boneless, skinless chicken breast. The cooking time is the same but cook the chicken until it reaches an internal temperature of 165°F.

Sheet Pan Trout *with* Brussels Sprouts and Potatoes

When you balance a meal—like in this dish—it provides your body the opportunity to take in a wider variety of nutrients needed for you to stay healthy.

PREP TIME 20 min // **COOK TIME** 32 min // **TOTAL TIME** 52 min // **SERVINGS** 4

SERVING SIZE 1 fillet + 1¼ cups vegetables

Meal Prep, One Pot/Pan | Vegetarian, Gluten-Free

Cooking spray

1 tablespoon extra-virgin olive oil

2 lemons, 1 juiced and 1 thinly sliced

2 cloves garlic, minced

2 tablespoons fresh dill, chopped

½ teaspoon kosher salt, divided

¼ teaspoon ground black pepper, divided

1 pound Brussels sprouts, trimmed and halved

1 pound baby potatoes

4 (6-ounce) fillets rainbow trout

4 teaspoons unsalted butter

4 fronds dill

1. Preheat the oven to 425°F. Coat a rimmed baking sheet with cooking spray.
2. In a large bowl, whisk together the oil, lemon juice, garlic, 2 tablespoons of chopped dill, ¼ teaspoon of the salt, and ⅛ teaspoon of the pepper. Add the Brussels sprouts and potatoes, and toss to evenly coat.
3. Gently pour the Brussels sprouts and potatoes onto the baking sheet in a single layer. Place in the preheated oven and roast until the vegetables begin to slightly brown, tossing halfway through, about 20 minutes.
4. Carefully remove the baking sheet from the oven, making room in the center of the baking sheet. Arrange the trout in the center of the baking sheet, moving the vegetables around it. Sprinkle the trout with the remaining ¼ teaspoon of the salt and ⅛ teaspoon of the pepper. Evenly distribute the lemon slices on the top of the trout. Top one lemon slice on each fillet with 1 teaspoon of butter and top each pat of butter with 1 frond of dill. Return the baking sheet to the oven and continue cooking until the trout reaches a minimum internal temperature of 145°F, 10 to 12 minutes.
5. *To serve:* On each of four plates, spoon one-quarter of the vegetables and 1 fillet of trout. Serve warm.

6. *To meal prep:* In each of four resealable containers, place one-quarter of the vegetables and 1 fillet. Cover and refrigerate for up to 4 days.
7. *To reheat*: Transfer the contents to a microwave-safe plate and microwave on high for 1½ minutes; let stand for 2 minutes to allow the heat to distribute evenly.

Nutrition Information (per serving): Calories 450; Total Fat 18g; Saturated Fat 6g; Protein 41g; Total Carbohydrates 31g; Fiber 6g; Total Sugars 3g (Includes Added Sugars 0g); Sodium 277mg

Toby's Tip: Swap the trout for salmon, arctic char, or snapper.

Creamy Salmon Ziti *with* Sun-Dried Tomatoes and Spinach

The trick to making this dish creamy without much artery-clogging saturated fat is by using reduced-fat ultra-filtered milk. The milk is thick and creamy on its own and adds a boatload of protein to the dish.

PREP TIME 15 min // **COOK TIME** 28 min // **TOTAL TIME** 43 min // **SERVINGS** 4 // **SERVING SIZE** 1¼ cups

Meal Prep, Freezer-Friendly | **Vegetarian**

- 8 ounces dry ziti pasta
- 1 cup frozen peas
- 3 tablespoons olive oil, divided
- 1 pound salmon fillet
- 2 cloves garlic, minced
- ¼ cup sun-dried tomatoes, roughly chopped
- 2 tablespoons all-purpose flour
- 2 cups 2 percent ultra-filtered milk (13 grams protein per 1 cup serving)
- 3 cups loosely packed spinach leaves, chopped
- ½ teaspoon kosher salt
- ¼ teaspoon ground black pepper
- ¼ cup fresh flat-leaf parsley leaves, chopped

1. Fill a medium saucepan three-quarters full with water and bring to a boil over high heat. Add the ziti, reduce the heat to medium, and simmer for 5 minutes. Add the peas and continue to simmer until the pasta is al dente, 5 to 7 minutes more. Drain and transfer the pasta to a large bowl. Set aside for 10 minutes to slightly cool.
2. Heat 2 tablespoons of the oil in a large skillet over medium heat. Once the oil is shimmering, add the salmon, skin-side down, and cook until the internal temperature reaches 145°F, 5 to 7 minutes per side. Transfer the salmon to a clean cutting board and allow to cool for 10 minutes. Remove the skin and cut the salmon into bite-size pieces.
3. In the same skillet, heat the remaining 1 tablespoon of the oil over medium heat. Once the oil is shimmering, add the garlic and cook until fragrant, about 1 minute. Add the tomatoes and cook until softened, about 1 minute. Sprinkle the flour over the vegetables and stir for 1 minute. Slowly add ¼ cup of the milk at a time, continuously whisking until the mixture thickens, about 8 minutes. Add the spinach, salt, and pepper, and cook until the spinach has wilted, about 1 minute. Add the salmon and peas and toss to evenly coat. Transfer the pasta to a serving bowl and garnish with the parsley.
4. *To serve:* In each of four bowls, spoon 1¾ cups of the pasta; enjoy warm.

5. *To meal prep:* In each of four resealable containers, spoon 1¾ cups of the pasta. Cover and refrigerate for up to 4 days or freeze for up to 2 months.
6. *To reheat:* To defrost, transfer to the refrigerator for 24 hours or up to 4 days. To reheat, transfer to a microwave-safe bowl and microwave on high for 1½ minutes; let stand for 2 minutes to allow the heat to distribute evenly.

Nutrition Information (per serving): Calories 439; Total Fat 19g; Saturated Fat 4g; Protein 27g; Total Carbohydrates 37g; Fiber 4g; Total Sugars 5g (Includes Added Sugars 0g); Sodium 243mg

Toby's Tip: Swap fresh salmon for the same amount of drained salmon canned in water.

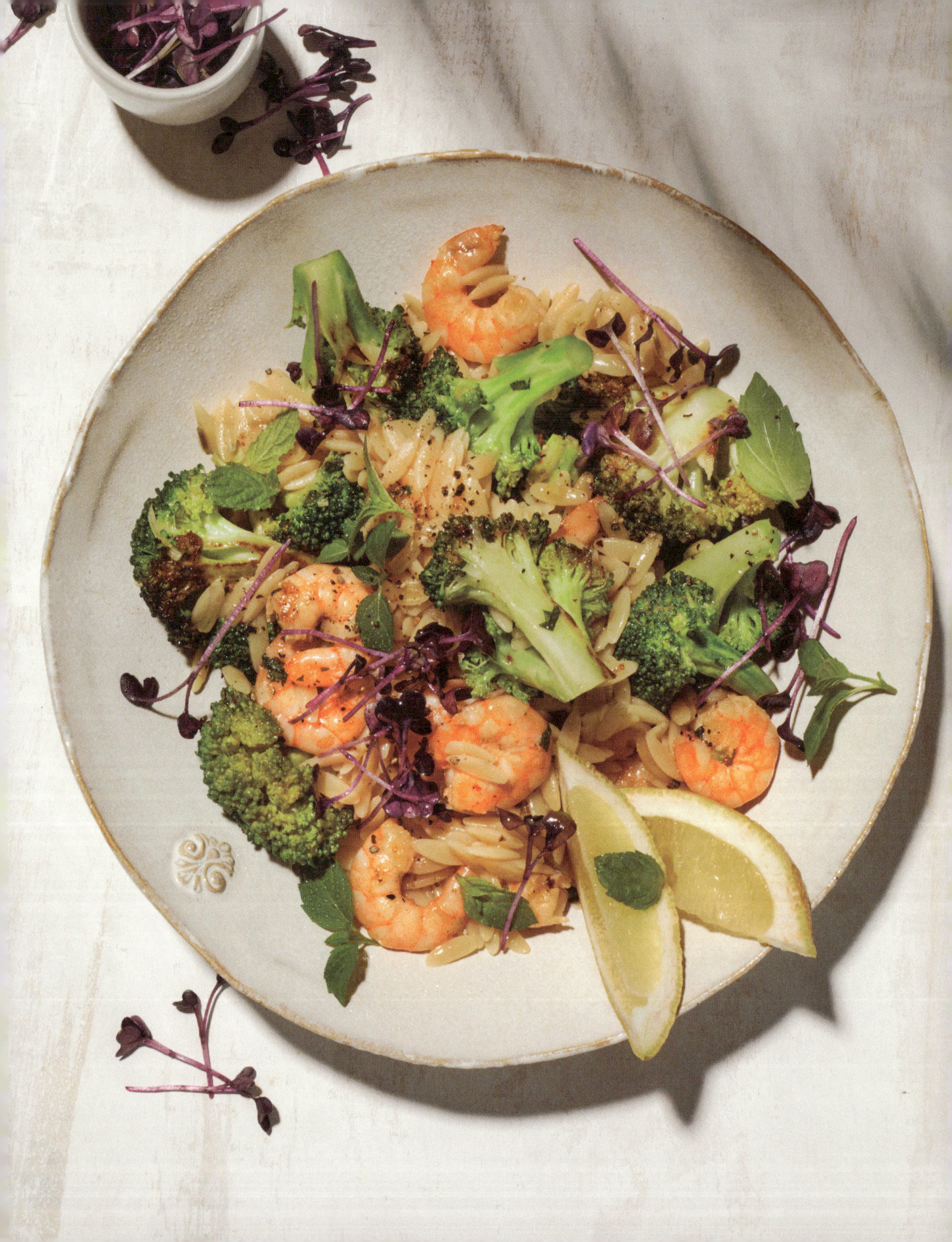

Lemon Shrimp *with* Orzo and Broccoli

This simple and light one-pot meal is perfect to whip up on a busy weeknight. Shrimp is a very lean protein, and while it does contain cholesterol, research shows that dietary cholesterol has little effect on blood cholesterol levels. So go on—enjoy your shrimp!

PREP TIME 15 min // **COOK TIME** 30 min // **TOTAL TIME** 45 min // **SERVINGS** 4 // **SERVING SIZE** 1¾ cups

Meal Prep, Freezer-Friendly | **Vegetarian**

FOR THE ORZO

1 cup dry orzo

2 cups low-sodium vegetable broth

FOR THE BROCCOLI

1 pound broccoli florets

FOR THE SHRIMP

1 pound shrimp, peeled and deveined

¼ teaspoon kosher salt

¼ teaspoon ground black pepper

2 tablespoons olive oil

2 tablespoons unsalted butter

1 small onion, chopped

2 cloves garlic, minced

TO ASSEMBLE THE DISH

½ cup low-sodium vegetable broth

Zest and juice of 1 lemon

3 tablespoons unsalted butter

1 clove garlic, minced

¼ teaspoon kosher salt

¼ teaspoon red pepper flakes

¼ cup fresh flat-leaf parsley leaves, chopped

¼ cup basil leaves, cut into ¼-inch ribbons

1 tablespoon Parmesan cheese, grated

1. *For the orzo:* Fill a medium saucepan three-quarters with water and bring to a boil over high heat. Add the orzo and broth, and return to a boil. Reduce the heat to medium-low and simmer, uncovered, until the orzo is tender, 10 minutes. Drain in a colander and allow to slightly cool for 10 minutes.
2. *For the broccoli:* Fill a medium saucepan with 2 inches of water. Fit with a steamer basket and bring to a boil over high heat. Add the broccoli, cover, and cook until the broccoli is slightly tender but still firm, 4 to 6 minutes. Transfer the broccoli to a separate colander and allow to slightly cool for 5 minutes.
3. *For the shrimp:* Season the shrimp with salt and pepper.
4. Heat the oil and butter in a large sauté pan over medium heat. Once the oil is shimmering, add the onion and garlic, and cook until the onion is translucent and the garlic is fragrant, about 2 minutes. Add the shrimp and cook, uncovered, until opaque, 5 to 6 minutes, turning once. Using a slotted spoon, transfer the shrimp to a large plate.

recipe continues 

5. *To assemble the dish:* In the same large sauté pan, combine the vegetable broth and lemon juice. Bring the mixture to a boil over high heat, then reduce the heat to medium and simmer until the liquid is reduced by half, 3 to 4 minutes. Add the zest, butter, garlic, salt, and red pepper flakes, and stir until the butter is melted, about 3 minutes. Add the orzo and broccoli and toss to evenly coat. Return the shrimp to the saucepan and toss to combine. Add the parsley, basil, and Parmesan, and stir to combine.
6. *To serve:* On each of four plates, spoon 1¾ cups of the shrimp and orzo; serve warm.
7. *To meal prep:* In each of four resealable containers, spoon 1¾ cups of the orzo. Cover and refrigerate for up to 4 days or freeze for up to 2 months. To defrost, transfer to the refrigerator for at least 24 hours or up to 4 days.
8. *To reheat*: Transfer to a microwave-safe plate and microwave on high for 1½ minutes; let stand for 2 minutes to allow the heat to distribute evenly.

Nutrition Information (per serving): Calories 435; Total Fat 17g; Saturated Fat 7g; Protein 32g; Total Carbohydrates 40g; Fiber 9g; Total Sugars 4g (Includes Added Sugars 0g); Sodium 460mg

Toby's Tip: Frozen (and defrosted) or fresh shrimp work equally well. To save time, buy your shrimp peeled and deveined.

Honey Garlic Salmon Bowls *with* Mango Salsa

Enjoy a symphony of flavors in every mouthful, where sweet honey harmonizes with savory salmon, brightened by notes of tangy mango.

PREP TIME 30 min // **COOK TIME** 25 min // **TOTAL TIME** 55 min // **SERVINGS** 4

SERVING SIZE 1 fillet + ⅔ cups rice + ½ cup salsa

Meal Prep | **Vegetarian, Gluten-Free, Dairy-Free**

FOR THE SALMON

2 tablespoons reduced-sodium soy sauce

2 tablespoons liquid honey

2 scallions, greens and whites, chopped

2 large cloves garlic, minced

3 tablespoons olive oil, divided

1 tablespoon unseasoned rice vinegar

½ teaspoon ground ginger

4 (5-ounce) salmon fillets

FOR THE MANGO SALSA

1 mango, peeled, pitted, and finely diced

½ red bell pepper, seeds and ribs removed, finely diced

¼ small red onion, chopped

½ jalapeño pepper, seeds and ribs removed

¼ cup fresh cilantro leaves, chopped

Juice of 2 limes

¼ teaspoon kosher salt

FOR THE RICE

⅔ cup dry basmati rice

1¼ cups unsweetened coconut milk (45 calories per 1 cup serving)

1 cup frozen edamame

1. *For the salmon:* In a large bowl, whisk together the soy sauce, honey, scallions, garlic, 1 tablespoon oil, rice vinegar, and ginger. Add the salmon and toss to evenly coat. Cover and refrigerate for at least 20 minutes or up to 4 hours.
2. *For the mango salsa:* In a medium bowl, toss together the mango, bell pepper, red onion, jalapeño, cilantro, lime juice, and salt. Place in the refrigerator for at least 20 minutes to allow flavors to meld.
3. *For the rice:* In a medium saucepan, bring the rice, milk, and edamame to a boil over high heat. Reduce the heat, cover, and cook until the rice is tender, 15 minutes. Fluff the rice with a fork.
4. *To finish the salmon:* Heat the remaining 2 tablespoons of oil in a large skillet over medium heat. Once the oil is shimmering, add the salmon, skin-side down, shaking off the excess marinade, and cook until the salmon reaches an internal temperature of 145°F, 4 to 5 minutes on each side. Transfer the salmon to a clean plate. Discard the marinade.

recipe continues 

5. *To serve:* In each of four bowls, add ⅔ cups of the rice and top with 1 fillet of salmon and about ½ cup of the salsa. Serve immediately.
6. *To meal prep:* In each of four containers, place ⅔ cup of rice and 1 salmon fillet. In each of four small containers, place ½ cup salsa. Cover the containers and refrigerate for 3 days.
7. *To reheat*: Transfer fish to a microwave-safe plate and microwave on high for 90 seconds; allow to stand for 2 minutes before topping with the salsa.

Nutrition Information (per serving): Calories 565; Total Fat 28g; Saturated Fat 7g; Protein 35g; Total Carbohydrates 47g; Fiber 3g; Total Sugars 16g (Includes Added Sugars 6.5g); Sodium 320mg

Toby's Tip: To save time, purchase store-bought mango salsa.

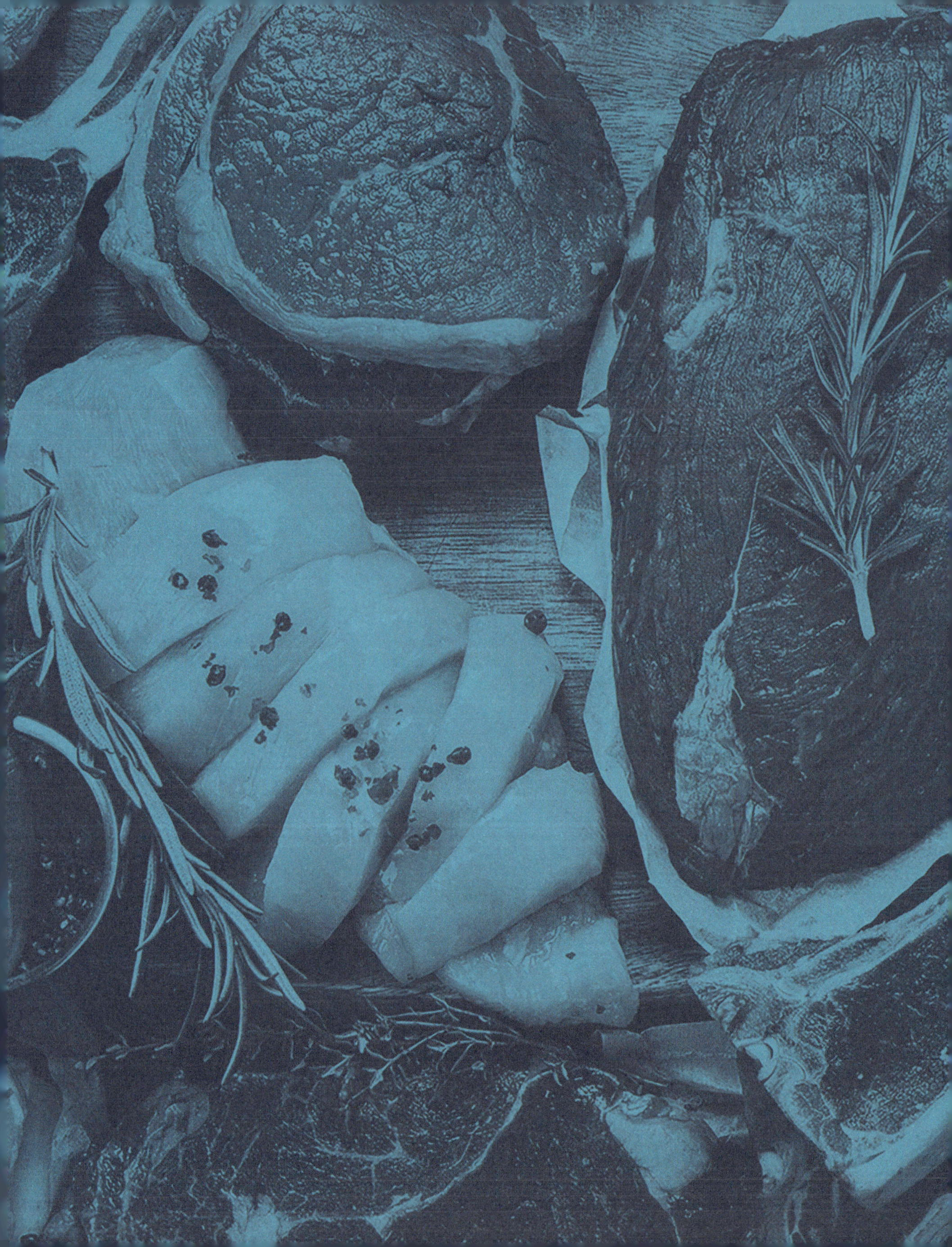

CHAPTER 9

Poultry and Meat Mains

Chicken Piccata over Angel Hair

A healthier take on a classic, this dish delivers 42 grams of protein and the same delicious taste, but with reduced saturated fat and sodium, making it heart healthy.

PREP TIME 20 min // **COOK TIME** 27 min // **TOTAL TIME** 47 min // **SERVINGS** 4

SERVING SIZE 1 cup pasta + ~4 ounces chicken with sauce

Meal Prep, Freezer-Friendly

- 8 ounces dried spaghetti (enriched white or whole wheat)
- 1⅓ pounds boneless, skinless chicken breasts, thinly sliced
- ½ teaspoon kosher salt, divided
- ½ teaspoon ground black pepper, divided
- ¼ cup + 2 teaspoons all-purpose flour, divided
- 1 teaspoon dried oregano
- ½ teaspoon onion powder
- ½ teaspoon garlic powder
- 3 tablespoons olive oil, divided
- 1 medium yellow onion, cut into ½-inch slices
- 1 clove garlic, minced
- ½ cup low-sodium chicken broth
- Juice of 1 lemon
- 2 tablespoons white cooking wine or dry white wine
- 2 tablespoons capers, drained
- 1 tablespoon fresh flat-leaf parsley leaves, chopped
- 1 tablespoon unsalted butter

1. Fill a large saucepan three-quarters full with water and bring to a boil over high heat. Stir in the spaghetti and cook, uncovered, until the spaghetti is al dente, about 10 minutes. Drain and set aside.
2. Sprinkle both sides of the chicken with ¼ teaspoon each of the salt and pepper.
3. In a medium bowl, sift together ¼ cup of the flour and the oregano, onion powder, and garlic powder. Dredge the chicken in the flour mixture, turning to coat.
4. Heat 2 tablespoons of the oil in a large sauté pan over medium heat. Once the oil is shimmering, add half the chicken and cook until the chicken is browned, about 2 minutes per side. Transfer the cooked chicken to a clean plate and repeat with the remaining chicken; set aside.
5. In the same pan, heat the remaining 1 tablespoon of oil over medium heat. Once the oil is shimmering, add the onion and garlic and cook until the onion is softened and garlic is fragrant, about 2 minutes. Whisk together the broth, lemon juice, and remaining 2 teaspoons of flour. Continue whisking until the sauce has slightly thickened and liquid is reduced, about 3 minutes. Whisk in the wine, capers, parsley, butter, and remaining ¼ teaspoon each of the salt and pepper until incorporated. Add the chicken, coat with the sauce, and continue cooking until the chicken reaches an internal temperature of 165°F, about 4 minutes.

6. *To serve*: On each of four plates place 1 cup of the cooked spaghetti and top with about 6 ounces of chicken breast and 2 to 3 tablespoons of the sauce. Serve warm.
7. *To meal prep:* In each of four resealable containers, place 1 cup of spaghetti and 1 chicken breast with 2 to 3 tablespoons of the sauce. Cover and refrigerate for up to 4 days or freeze for up to 2 months.
8. *To reheat:* To defrost, transfer to the refrigerator overnight. To reheat, transfer onto a microwave-safe plate and microwave on high for 90 seconds. Let stand for 2 minutes to allow the heat to distribute evenly.

Nutrition Information (per serving): Calories 553; Total Fat 18g; Saturated Fat 4g; Protein 42g; Total Carbohydrates 52g; Fiber 3g; Total Sugars 3g (Includes Added Sugars 0g); Sodium 341mg

Toby's Tip: To make this dish dairy-free, omit the butter.

Tomato-Basil Chicken Thighs and Rice

This one-pot meal was a fixture of my kids' childhood, frequently requested by them and their friends. Thanks to all the time they spent with me in the kitchen, they've become confident cooks who can now prepare this dish on their own.

PREP TIME 20 min // **COOK TIME** 37 min // **TOTAL TIME** 57 min // **SERVINGS** 4
SERVING SIZE 2 cups (including chicken)

Meal Prep, Freezer-Friendly, One Pot/Pan | Gluten-Free, Dairy-Free

1½ pounds boneless, skinless chicken thighs
½ teaspoon kosher salt, divided
½ teaspoon ground black pepper, divided
2 tablespoons olive oil, divided
1 medium yellow onion, chopped
1 medium red bell pepper, seeds and ribs removed, chopped
2 cloves garlic, minced
1 cup dry white basmati rice
1½ cups low-sodium chicken broth
1 (14.5-ounce) can fire-roasted diced tomatoes, with juice
1 cup cherry tomatoes, halved
1 tablespoon balsamic vinegar
¼ teaspoon red pepper flakes
¼ cup basil leaves, cut into ¼-inch ribbons

1. Sprinkle the chicken with ¼ teaspoon each of the salt and pepper.
2. Heat 1 tablespoon of the oil in a large skillet over a medium-high heat. Once the oil is shimmering, add the chicken and cook until browned, 3 to 4 minutes on each side. Transfer the chicken to a clean plate; set aside.
3. Heat the remaining 1 tablespoon of the oil in the same skillet over medium heat. Once the oil is shimmering, add the onion, peppers, and garlic, and cook until the vegetables are softened and garlic is fragrant, about 4 minutes.
4. Add the rice, chicken broth, diced tomatoes, cherry tomatoes, balsamic vinegar, red pepper flakes, and remaining ¼ teaspoon each of the salt and pepper; stir to combine. Return the chicken thighs to the pan and nestle within the rice. Increase the heat to high and bring the mixture to a boil. Reduce the heat to medium-low, cover, and simmer for about 25 minutes, stirring occasionally, until the rice is tender and chicken has reached a minimum internal temperature of 165°F.
5. Remove the skillet from the heat and stir in the basil leaves.
6. *To serve:* On each of four plates, spoon 2 cups of the mixture. Enjoy warm.

7. *To meal prep:* In each of four resealable containers, spoon 2 cups of the chicken and rice mixture. Cover and refrigerate for up to 4 days or freeze for up to 2 months.

8. *To reheat:* To defrost, transfer to the refrigerator overnight. To reheat, transfer to a microwave-safe plate and microwave on high for 2 minutes.

Nutrition Information (per serving): Calories 481; Total Fat 14g; Saturated Fat 3g; Protein 39g; Total Carbohydrates 49g; Fiber 4g; Total Sugars 6g (Includes Added Sugars 0g); Sodium 540mg

Toby's Tip: Swap the chicken thighs for skinless chicken tenderloins or boneless, skinless chicken breasts cut into pieces.

Chicken Ramen Bowls

Ramen is a trendy meal for my young adult kids. This homemade version lets you control the ingredients. While there are carbs from the ramen noodles, the 2-ounce portions keep them in check and allows room for more delicious vegetables.

PREP TIME 25 min // **COOK TIME** 16 min // **TOTAL TIME** 41 min // **SERVINGS** 4 // **SERVING SIZE** 1 bowl

Meal Prep | **Dairy-free**

4 large eggs

2 cups (8 ounces) rotisserie chicken, skin removed, shredded

8 ounces dried ramen noodles

1 tablespoon sesame oil

1½ piece fresh ginger, chopped

2 cloves garlic, minced

1 (5-ounce) container shiitake mushrooms, thinly sliced

6 cups low-sodium chicken broth

2 tablespoons reduced-sodium soy sauce

1 teaspoon unseasoned rice vinegar

1 teaspoon sriracha-style hot sauce

1 pound bok choy, leaves and stems, roughly chopped

1 cup frozen shelled edamame

½ cup sprouts of choice

1 medium carrot, peeled and shredded

2 medium scallions, chopped

1 jalapeño pepper, seeds and ribs removed, thinly sliced

1. Place the eggs in a medium saucepan and cover with cold water. Place the saucepan over high heat and bring to a boil; cook for 3 minutes. Remove the saucepan from the heat, cover, and allow to stand for 10 minutes. Drain, and run cold water over the eggs until completely cool, about 10 minutes. Once cooled, peel the eggs and cut in half lengthwise.
2. Fill a large saucepan three-quarters full with water and bring to a boil over high heat. Add the ramen noodles and cook until al dente, about 3 minutes. Drain the noodles in a colander and set aside.
3. In a separate large saucepan, heat the oil over medium heat. Once the oil is shimmering, add the ginger and garlic, and cook until fragrant, about 90 seconds. Add the mushrooms and continue cooking until slightly softened, about 3 minutes. Add the broth, soy sauce, rice vinegar, and sriracha, cover, and bring to a boil over high heat. Reduce the heat to medium-low and add the bok choy and edamame. Cook, uncovered, until the bok choy is wilted, about 5 minutes.
4. *To serve:* In each of four bowls, add 1 cup of the ramen noodles, ½ cup chicken, 2 egg halves, 2 tablespoons sprouts, and one-quarter of the carrots and scallions. Pour about 2 cups of the broth over the bowl. Garnish with an even amount of jalapeño.
5. *To meal prep:* In each of four resealable containers, place the contents of the bowls. Cover and store in the refrigerator for up to 4 days.

6. *To reheat*: Transfer to a microwave-safe bowl and microwave on high for 2 minutes; let sit for 2 minutes to allow the heat to distribute evenly.

Nutrition Information (per serving): Calories 483; Total Fat 12g; Saturated Fat 3g; Protein 32g; Total Carbohydrates 60g; Fiber 4g; Total Sugars 6g (Includes Added Sugars 0g); Sodium 651mg

Toby's Tip: Use leftover chicken pieces instead of the rotisserie chicken to help minimize food waste and creatively reuse leftovers.

Chicken "Fried" Rice *with* Vegetables

Give this dish a try and it's sure to become a regular fixture in your dinner rotation. The deeply satisfying Asian-inspired flavors, rich with savory and umami notes, make it a guaranteed favorite.

PREP TIME 20 min // **COOK TIME** 47 min // **TOTAL TIME** 1 hour, 7 min // **SERVINGS** 4 // **SERVING SIZE** 2 cups

Meal Prep, Freezer-Friendly | Dairy-free

- 1 cup dry brown rice
- 3 cups low-sodium chicken broth
- 1 cup frozen shelled edamame
- 12 ounces boneless, skinless chicken breast, cut into ½-inch pieces
- ¼ teaspoon kosher salt
- ⅛ teaspoon ground black pepper
- 3 tablespoons olive oil, divided
- ¼ cup reduced-sodium soy sauce
- 2 teaspoons liquid honey
- ¼ teaspoon ground ginger
- 1 small yellow onion, chopped
- 1 red bell pepper, seeds and ribs removed, chopped
- 1 medium carrot, peeled and shredded
- 3 large eggs, beaten
- 2 scallions, whites and greens, sliced

1. In a medium pot, bring the rice, edamame, and water to a boil over high heat. Reduce the heat to medium-low, cover, and simmer, stirring occasionally, until tender, about 30 minutes. Fluff with a fork; set aside.
2. Sprinkle the chicken with salt and pepper.
3. Heat 2 tablespoons of oil in a large sauté pan over medium heat. Once the oil is shimmering, add the chicken and cook on all sides until the internal temperature is 165°F, about 6 minutes. Transfer the chicken to a clean plate; set aside.
4. In a small bowl, whisk together the soy sauce, liquid honey, and ginger.
5. Heat the remaining 1 tablespoon of the oil in a large sauté pan over medium heat. Once the oil is shimmering, add the onion, pepper, and carrots, and cook until softened, 4 minutes. Push the vegetables aside and add the beaten eggs. Cook the eggs to a scramble, 2 to 3 minutes, and then mix with the vegetables. Add the cooked rice and combine with the pieces of egg. Add the cooked chicken, soy sauce mixture, and scallions, and toss to combine. Continue cooking for 3 to 4 minutes to allow the flavors to meld.
6. *To serve:* On each of four plates, spoon 2 cups of the rice mixture; serve warm.
7. *To meal prep:* In each of four resealable containers, spoon 2 cups of the rice mixture. Cover and refrigerate for up to 4 days or freeze for up to 2 months.

8. *To reheat:* To defrost, place overnight in the refrigerator. To reheat, transfer to a microwave-safe plate and microwave on high for about 90 seconds; let stand 2 minutes for the heat to distribute evenly.

Nutrition Information (per serving): Calories 519; Total Fat 20g; Saturated Fat 4g; Protein 34g; Total Carbohydrates 51g; Fiber 4g; Total Sugars 9g (Includes Added Sugars 4g); Sodium 653mg

Toby's Tip: Swap the chicken for the same amount of salmon. Cook in a preheated 425°F oven for 12 to 14 minutes, until the fish reaches an internal temperature of 145°F.

Chicken Stir-Fry *with* Broccoli, Snow Peas, and Mushrooms

Featuring a delicate sauce of chicken broth and white wine, this stir-fry offers a subtle, sophisticated flavor. It's a delicious, lower-sodium alternative that doesn't compromise on taste.

PREP TIME 30 Min // **COOK TIME** 38 Min // **TOTAL TIME** 1 hour, 8 min // **SERVINGS** 4

SERVING SIZE 1¾ cups of stir-fry + ¾ cup rice

Meal Prep, Freezer-Friendly | **Dairy-free**

FOR THE RICE

2 cups water

1 cup dry Jasmine rice

FOR THE WHITE SAUCE

1 tablespoon olive oil

1 small onion, chopped

2 cloves garlic, minced

1¾ cups low-sodium chicken broth, divided

1 cup white cooking wine or dry white wine

2 teaspoons cornstarch

1 teaspoon dried thyme

1 teaspoon dried parsley

¼ teaspoon kosher salt

1 tablespoon unsalted butter

FOR THE STIR-FRY

1 pound boneless, skinless chicken breast, cut into bite-size pieces

¼ teaspoon kosher salt

⅛ teaspoon ground black pepper

2 tablespoons olive oil, divided

2 cups broccoli florets

1 (8-ounce) container white button mushrooms, sliced

1 cup snow peas, trimmed

1. *For the rice:* In a medium saucepan, add the water and rice and bring to a boil over high heat. Reduce the heat to medium-low, cover, and simmer until the rice is tender, about 15 minutes. Fluff with a fork and set aside.
2. *For the sauce:* Heat the oil in a medium skillet over medium heat. Once the oil is shimmering, add the onion and garlic, and cook until the onion is soft and translucent and garlic is fragrant, about 3 minutes. Add 1½ cups of the broth and wine and bring to a boil over high heat. Reduce the heat to medium-low and simmer, whisking occasionally, until about one-third of the liquid is reduced, 10 to 12 minutes.

3. In a small bowl, whisk together the remaining ¼ cup broth and cornstarch until the mixture is slightly thickened, about 1 minute. Whisk in the cornstarch mixture and cook until the mixture has thickened, 4 to 5 minutes. Whisk in the thyme, parsley, and salt until combined. Add the butter, and whisk until melted and sauce is glistening. Remove the skillet from the heat and set aside.
4. *For the stir-fry:* Sprinkle the chicken with the salt and pepper.
5. Heat 1 tablespoon of the oil in a large wok over high heat. Once the oil is shimmering, add the chicken and cook, turning on each side, until the chicken is cooked through, about 8 minutes. Transfer the chicken to a clean plate.
6. In the same large wok, heat the remaining 1 tablespoon of oil. Once the oil is shimmering, add the broccoli and mushrooms, and cook until the vegetables are slightly soft, about 6 minutes. Add the snow peas and cook until slightly softened, about 3 minutes. Add the cooked chicken and sauce and toss to evenly coat.
7. *To serve:* On each of four plates, spoon ¾ cup of rice and top with 1¾ cups of the stir-fry. Serve warm.
8. *To meal prep:* In each of four resealable containers, spoon ¾ cups of rice and 1¾ cups of the stir-fry. Cover and refrigerate for up to 4 days or freeze for up to 2 months.
9. *To reheat:* To defrost, transfer to the refrigerator overnight or up to 4 days. To reheat, transfer to a small saucepan and bring the sauce to a boil over high heat, and then reduce the heat and cook until heated through, about 5 minutes. Alternatively, transfer the stir-fry and rice to a microwave-safe plate and microwave on high for 1½ minutes; let stand for 2 minutes to allow the heat to distribute evenly.

Nutrition Information (per serving): Calories [illegible]; Total Fat [illegible]; Saturated Fat [illegible]; Protein 33g; Total Carbohydrates 47g; Fiber 2g; Total Sugars 4g (Includes Added Sugars 0g); Sodium 291mg

Toby's Tip: Stir-fries are my favorite way to use leftover vegetables in the refrigerator, reduce food waste, and stretch my food dollar. Substitute veggies like cauliflower, string beans, peppers, zucchini, carrots, or whatever you have on hand.

Sheet Pan Herbed Turkey Breast *with* String Beans and Cranberries

These days my Thanksgiving feast is a more intimate gathering. Instead of buying a huge turkey that takes hours to prepare and cook, I opt for turkey breasts and flavor them with a variety of herbs. I then fill the rest of my plate with delicious veggies and tart cranberries. It's a satisfying and mouthwatering meal that doesn't take hours to cook up.

PREP TIME 35 min // **COOK TIME** 55 min // **TOTAL TIME** 1 hour, 30 min // **SERVINGS** 4

SERVING SIZE about 5 ounces turkey + ¾ cup string beans

Meal Prep, One Pot/Pan | **Gluten-Free, Dairy-Free**

- Nonstick cooking spray
- 1½ teaspoons sweet paprika
- 1 teaspoon dried rosemary
- ¾ teaspoon kosher salt, divided
- ½ teaspoon garlic powder
- ½ teaspoon ground sage
- ¼ teaspoon ground black pepper, divided
- 2 tablespoons unsalted butter, softened
- 1 (1½-pound) boneless, skin-on split turkey breast
- 1 pound green beans, trimmed
- 2 tablespoons extra-virgin olive oil
- ½ cup dried unsweetened cranberries
- 1 teaspoon dried parsley
- 1 teaspoon dried oregano

1. Preheat the oven to 425°F. Coat a rimmed baking sheet with nonstick cooking spray.
2. In a small bowl, add the sweet paprika, rosemary, ½ teaspoon salt, garlic powder, sage, and ⅛ teaspoon of the pepper; mix to combine.
3. Using clean hands, spread the butter over all sides of the turkey, and then rub the spice mixture over the turkey. Place the turkey, skin-side up, on the prepared baking sheet and coat the top of the turkey with nonstick cooking spray.
4. Roast the turkey in the preheated oven, uncovered, until the top is browned, 15 to 20 minutes.
5. While the turkey is roasting, prepare the green beans and place in a large bowl. Add the oil, cranberries, parsley, oregano, and the remaining ¼ teaspoon of salt and ⅛ teaspoon of pepper; toss to combine.

6. Loosely cover the turkey with aluminum foil and continue cooking for 15 minutes. Carefully remove the sheet pan from the oven and transfer the green beans onto the baking sheet, arranging them in a single layer around the covered turkey. Return the sheet pan to the oven and continue cooking until the internal temperature of the turkey reaches 165°F and the green beans are browned, 15 to 20 minutes. Remove the sheet pan from the oven and carefully remove the aluminum foil and discard. Allow the turkey to rest for 20 minutes before slicing.
7. *To serve:* On each of six plates, place about 5 ounces of turkey and ¾ cup of string beans. Enjoy warm.
8. *To meal prep:* In each of six resealable containers, place 5 ounces turkey and ¾ cup string beans. Cover and refrigerate for up to 4 days.
9. *To reheat*: Transfer to a microwave-safe plate and microwave on high for 1½ minutes. Let stand for 2 minutes to allow the heat to evenly distribute.

Nutrition Information (per serving): Calories 448; Total Fat 23g; Saturated Fat 8g; Protein 40g; Total Carbohydrates 19g; Fiber 4g; Total Sugars 14g (Includes Added Sugars 9g); Sodium 303mg

Toby's Tip: Turkey breast isn't always available year-round. Boneless, skinless chicken breasts with rib meat can be substituted and works perfectly!

Skillet Ground Beef *with* Sweet Potatoes

This one-pot meal is one of my favorites to have as leftovers for lunch the next day. Fair warning: If you bring it to work and reheat it, your officemates will be asking for a taste.

PREP TIME 20 min // **COOK TIME** 37 min // **TOTAL TIME** 57 min // **SERVINGS** 6 // **SERVING SIZE** 1¼ cups

Meal Prep, Freezer-Friendly, One Pot/Pan | Gluten-Free

- ½ teaspoon chipotle chili powder
- ½ teaspoon smoked paprika
- ½ teaspoon ground cumin
- ½ teaspoon ground oregano
- ½ teaspoon ground coriander
- ¼ teaspoon kosher salt
- ⅛ teaspoon ground black pepper
- 3 tablespoons olive or avocado oil, divided
- 1 medium yellow onion, chopped
- 1 clove garlic, minced
- 1 pound ground beef (at least 90 percent lean)
- 2 medium (about 1¼ pounds) sweet potatoes, peeled and diced in 1-inch cubes
- 1 (14.5-ounce) can fire-roasted diced tomatoes, drained
- 1 (4-ounce) can diced green chilies, with liquids
- ⅓ cup water
- ½ cup reduced-fat shredded cheddar cheese

1. In a small bowl, mix together the chili powder, paprika, cumin, oregano, coriander, salt, and pepper; set aside.
2. Heat 2 tablespoons oil in a large sauté pan over medium heat. When the oil is shimmering, add the onion and garlic, and cook until the onion is soft and translucent and the garlic is fragrant, about 3 minutes. Add the ground beef and spice mixture, and cook, tossing occasionally, until the beef reaches a minimum internal temperature of 155°F, about 8 minutes. Transfer the beef to a clean plate and set aside.
3. Wipe the inside of the pan with a paper towel. Place the pan over medium heat and add the remaining 1 tablespoon of oil. Once the oil is shimmering, add the sweet potatoes and cook until slightly browned on all sides, about 5 minutes. Add the spice mixture, diced tomatoes, green chilies, and water, and bring to a boil over high heat. Reduce the heat to medium-low and simmer, covered, until the potatoes are tender, about 20 minutes. Add the cooked ground beef and toss to combine. Sprinkle with the cheese, cover, and cook until the cheese has melted, about 1 minute. Serve warm.
4. *To serve:* On each of six plates, spoon 1¼ cups of the beef mixture. Serve warm.

5. *To meal prep:* In each of six resealable containers, spoon 1¼ cups of the beef mixture. Cover and refrigerate for up to 4 days or freeze for up to 2 months.
6. *To reheat:* To defrost, transfer to the refrigerator overnight or up to 4 days. To reheat, transfer to a microwave-safe plate and microwave on high for 2 minutes; let stand for 2 minutes to allow the heat to distribute evenly. Alternatively, transfer to a small saucepan with 1 tablespoon of water and bring to a boil over high heat. Reduce the heat to medium-low, cover, and cook for 5 minutes until heated through.

Nutrition Information (per serving): Calories 422; Total Fat 24g; Saturated Fat 8g; Protein 29g; Total Carbohydrates 20g; Fiber 4g; Total Sugars 6g (Includes Added Sugars 0g); Sodium 593mg

Toby's Tip: Swap the ground beef for ground turkey.

Beef and Bulgur Stuffed Peppers

Growing up, my grandmother Hannah used to make traditional stuffed peppers with ground beef, rice, and tomato sauce regularly. This recipe offers a delicious new take, with bulgur wheat at its heart and a medley of aromatic vegetables and spices.

PREP TIME 20 min // **COOK TIME** 54 min // **TOTAL TIME** 1 hour, 14 min // **SERVINGS** 4

SERVING SIZE 2 pepper halves

Meal Prep

- 1 cup water
- ½ cup dry bulgur
- Nonstick cooking spray
- 4 medium green bell peppers
- 1 tablespoon olive oil
- 1 small onion, chopped
- 1 clove garlic, minced
- 1 stalk celery, chopped
- 1 medium carrot, chopped
- ¾ pound ground beef (at least 90 percent lean)
- 2 tablespoons tomato paste
- ½ teaspoon ground coriander
- ½ teaspoon dried parsley
- ½ teaspoon ground paprika
- ½ teaspoon ground cumin
- ¼ teaspoon kosher salt
- ⅛ teaspoon ground allspice
- ⅛ teaspoon cayenne
- 8 tablespoons shredded Parmesan cheese, divided

1. Add the water and bulgur to a medium saucepan and bring to a boil over high heat. Reduce the heat to medium-low and simmer, covered, until the bulgur is tender, about 15 minutes. Fluff with a fork and allow to slightly cool, about 10 minutes.
2. Preheat the oven to 350°F. Coat a rimmed baking sheet with nonstick cooking spray.
3. Cut the peppers in half from the top down and remove the seeds and ribs. Place on the prepared baking sheet cup-side up.
4. Heat the oil in a large sauté pan over medium heat. Once the oil is shimmering, add the onion and garlic, and cook until the onion is soft and translucent and the garlic is fragrant, about 3 minutes. Add the celery and carrots, and sauté until softened, about 3 minutes. Add the ground beef and cook, breaking up the meat with a wooden spoon, until browned on all sides, about 8 minutes. Add the cooked bulgur, tomato paste, coriander, parsley, paprika, cumin, salt, allspice, and cayenne. Cook until warmed through, about 3 minutes.
5. Spoon the mixture into each pepper and, using clean hands, gently press down so the mixture is set inside. Arrange the peppers in the baking dish, spacing them about 1 inch apart. Top each pepper with 1 tablespoon Parmesan cheese. Cover the sheet pan loosely with aluminum foil.

6. Bake in the preheated oven until the peppers are soft and cheese has melted, 20 to 25 minutes. Remove the baking dish from the oven and set aside to slightly cool, about 15 minutes.

7. *To serve:* On each of four plates, place 2 pepper halves; serve warm.

8. *To meal prep:* In each of four resealable containers, place 2 pepper halves. Cover and refrigerate for up to 4 days.

9. *To reheat*: Transfer to a microwave-safe plate and microwave on high for 2 minutes. Let stand 2 minutes to allow the heat to distribute evenly.

Nutrition Information (per serving): Calories 346; Total Fat 16g; Saturated Fat 6g; Protein 26g; Total Carbohydrates 26g; Fiber 8g; Total Sugars 6g (Includes Added Sugars 0g); Sodium 397mg

Toby's Tip: To make the dish dairy-free, swap the Parmesan cheese for 8 teaspoons nutritional yeast.

Herbed Butter Steak *with* Broccoli Mashed Potatoes

When most people think about protein, a hearty steak comes to mind. In restaurants, steak is typically served with potatoes and broccoli, but this version combines the two, so you'll find chopped pieces of broccoli mixed within the red potato mash.

PREP TIME 45 min // **COOK TIME** 1 hour, 11 min // **TOTAL TIME** 1 hour, 56 min // **SERVINGS** 4

SERVING SIZE 1 steak + 1 cup mashed potatoes

Meal Prep | **Gluten-Free**

FOR THE STEAK

3 tablespoons extra-virgin olive oil

1 tablespoon balsamic vinegar

2 cloves garlic, minced

½ teaspoon dried rosemary

½ teaspoon dried oregano

½ teaspoon kosher salt

⅛ teaspoon ground black pepper

4 (6-ounce) sirloin steaks

1 tablespoon unsalted butter

FOR THE BROCCOLI MASHED POTATOES

Nonstick cooking spray

2 pounds (about 4 medium) Yukon Gold potatoes (with skin)

1½ cups broccoli, roughly chopped

Ice cubes

⅓ cup reduced-fat (2 percent) ultra-filtered milk (at least 13 grams protein per cup)

1 tablespoon unsalted butter

1 teaspoon dried chives

¼ teaspoon kosher salt

⅛ teaspoon ground black pepper

⅛ teaspoon garlic powder

1. *For the steak:* In a large bowl, whisk together the oil, balsamic vinegar, garlic, rosemary, oregano, salt, and pepper. Add the steaks and toss to evenly coat. Cover and refrigerate for at least 30 minutes or up to 24 hours.
2. *For the broccoli mashed potatoes:* Preheat the oven to 400°F. Coat a rimmed baking sheet with cooking spray.
3. Using a fork, poke several holes in the potatoes. Place the potatoes onto the prepared baking sheet and bake until fork tender, about 1 hour. Remove the sheet pan from the oven and allow potatoes to cool, about 15 minutes.
4. Increase the heat in the oven to 425°F.

5. While the potatoes are cooking, fill a medium saucepan with 1 inch of water and fit with a steamer basket. Bring the water to a boil over high heat. Add the broccoli, cover, and steam for 5 minutes. Working quickly, transfer the broccoli to a colander filled with ice cubes.
6. Transfer the potatoes to a large bowl and, using a potato masher, partially mash the potatoes. Add the milk, butter, chives, salt, pepper, and garlic powder, and mix to combine. Fold in the broccoli until evenly distributed.
7. *For the steaks:* Heat butter in a large cast-iron skillet or oven-safe skillet over medium-high heat. Once the butter is shimmering, add the steaks and cook, undisturbed, until browned, 2 to 3 minutes. Using tongs, flip the steak and brown on the other side, 2 to 3 minutes.
8. Carefully transfer the skillet to the preheated oven and cook until the steaks reach a minimum internal temperature of 145°F, 5 to 10 minutes (depending on the thickness of the steaks).
9. Carefully remove the skillet from the oven and transfer the steaks to a cutting board. Allow the steaks to rest so the juices distribute evenly, 10 minutes.
10. *To serve:* On each of four plates, place 1 steak, spooning the sauce from the pan over the top. Add 1 cup of the mashed potatoes alongside. Enjoy warm.
11. *To meal prep:* In each of four resealable containers, place 1 steak with sauce and 1 cup of mashed potatoes. Cover and refrigerate for up to 4 days.
12. *To reheat:* Transfer to a microwave-safe plate and microwave on high for 2 minutes. Let stand for 2 minutes to allow the heat to distribute evenly.

Nutrition Information (per serving): Calories 564; Total Fat 22g; Saturated Fat 8g; Protein 46g; Total Carbohydrates 44g; Fiber 4g; Total Sugars 2g (includes Added Sugars 0g); Sodium 329mg

Toby's Tip: To stretch your food dollar, buy sirloin steaks in bulk at your local warehouse club and freeze.

Poultry and Meat Mains

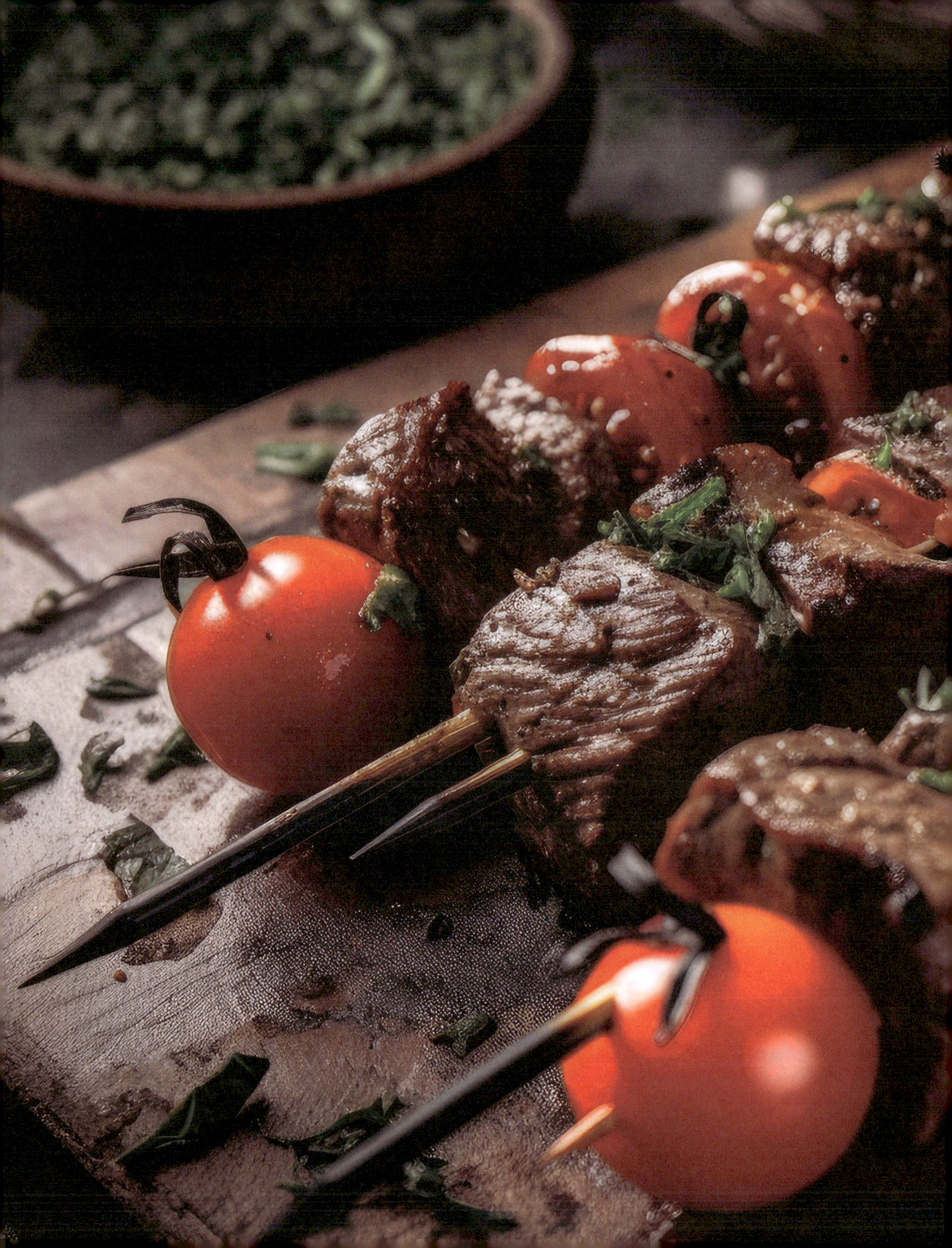

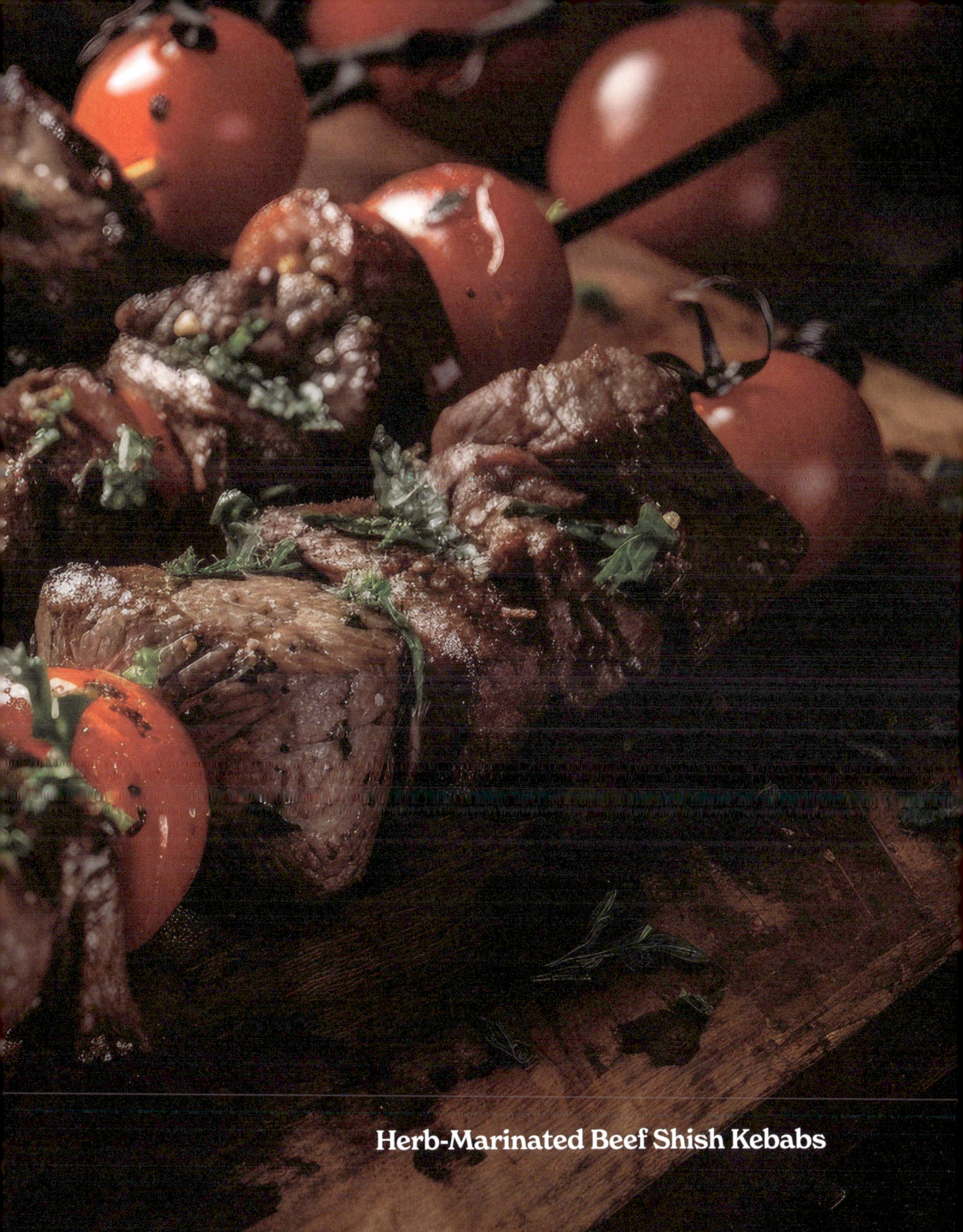

Herb-Marinated Beef Shish Kebabs

Herb-Marinated Beef Shish Kebabs

These Mediterranean-inspired kebabs feature a refreshing marinade made with olive oil, red wine vinegar, and herb sauce. It's a perfectly simple dish for weeknight dinners yet also fancy enough to serve guests.

PREP TIME 50 min // **COOK TIME** 12 min // **TOTAL TIME** 1 hour, 2 min // **SERVINGS** 4

SERVING SIZE 2 skewers

Meal Prep | **Gluten-Free, Dairy-Free**

½ cup olive oil

¼ cup red wine vinegar

Juice of 1 lemon

2 cloves garlic, minced

1 teaspoon dried rosemary

1 teaspoon dried thyme

1 teaspoon dried basil

1 teaspoon dried oregano

1 teaspoon dried marjoram

½ teaspoon ground sage

½ teaspoon kosher salt

⅛ teaspoon ground black pepper

1½ pounds beef sirloin (like top sirloin), cut into 2-inch cubes

Nonstick cooking spray (if using grill pan)

16 cherry tomatoes

16 (12-inch-long) skewers

1. In a large bowl, whisk together the oil, vinegar, lemon juice, garlic, rosemary, thyme, basil, oregano, marjoram, sage, salt, and pepper. Add the beef cubes and toss to coat evenly. Cover the bowl with plastic wrap and set in the refrigerator to marinate for at least 20 minutes or up to 24 hours.
2. If you are using wooden skewers, soak them in water for at least 10 minutes.
3. Preheat a grill or a grill pan over medium-high heat. If using a grill, brush with 1 tablespoon oil. If using a grill pan, coat with nonstick cooking spray.
4. Remove the beef from the marinade, allowing the excess to drip off; discard the marinade. Thread each skewer with 2 to 3 pieces of the beef and 2 tomatoes in an alternating pattern. Grill the kebabs, turning them several times until the beef is browned and reaches a minimum internal temperature is 145°F, about 12 minutes.
5. *To serve:* On each of 4 plates, place 2 meat skewers. Serve warm.
6. *To meal prep*: Into each of four containers, remove the meat and vegetables from 2 kebabs. Cover and refrigerate for up to 4 days or store in the freezer for up to 2 months.

7. *To reheat*: To defrost, transfer overnight to the refrigerator. To reheat, transfer to a microwave-safe plate and microwave on high for 2 minutes. Let stand for 2 minutes to allow the heat to distribute evenly.

Nutrition Information (per serving): Calories 490; Total Fat 39g; Saturated Fat 10g; Protein 30g; Total Carbohydrates 4g; Fiber 1g; Total Sugars 2g (Includes Added Sugars 0g); Sodium 190mg

Toby's Tip: Swap the beef for lamb. Serve either version with Couscous with Chickpeas, Peas, and Carrots on page 255.

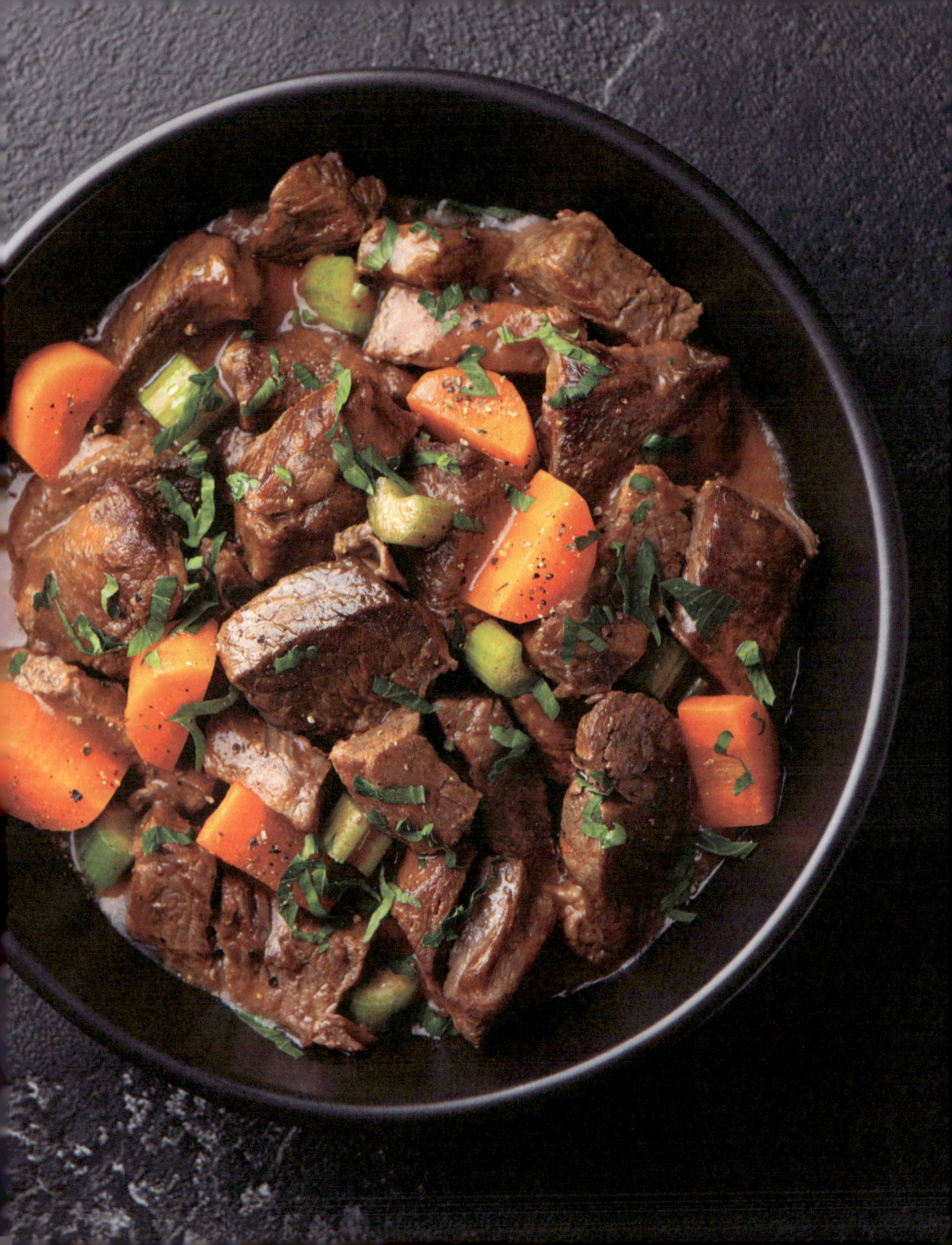

Comforting Beef Stew

There's nothing better on a cold night than a warming bowl of beef stew full of protein and vegetables. Serve with a crusty piece of bread for dipping to enjoy every last drop of the sauce.

PREP TIME 20 min // **COOK TIME** 1 hour, 31 min // **TOTAL TIME** 1 hour, 51 min // **SERVINGS** 4

SERVING SIZE 1¾ cups

Meal Prep, Freezer-Friendly, One Pot/Pan | **Dairy-free**

- 1¼ pounds boneless beef rounds, cut into ½-inch cubes
- ½ teaspoon kosher salt, divided
- ¼ teaspoon ground black pepper, divided
- 3 tablespoons olive oil, divided
- 1 medium yellow onion, chopped
- 2 stalks celery, chopped
- 2 cloves garlic, minced
- 2 tablespoons all-purpose flour
- 1 teaspoon ground paprika
- 1 teaspoon dried thyme
- 1 teaspoon dried oregano
- 2 cups low-sodium beef broth or water, divided
- 2 tablespoons tomato paste
- 2 medium carrots, cut into 1-inch rounds

1. Sprinkle the beef with ¼ teaspoon of the salt and ⅛ teaspoon of the pepper.
2. In a large pot, heat 2 tablespoons of the oil over medium heat. Once the oil is shimmering, add the beef and cook on all sides until browned, about 8 minutes. Transfer the beef to a clean plate.
3. Heat the remaining 1 tablespoon of the oil in the same pot. Once the oil is shimmering, add the onion, celery, and garlic, and cook until the vegetables are translucent and garlic is fragrant, about 5 minutes. Sprinkle the flour, paprika, thyme, and oregano over the vegetables and cook, stirring, for 1 minute. Add 1 cup of the broth, and cook, stirring occasionally, until the mixture has thickened, 1 to 2 minutes. Add the remaining 1 cup of the broth, tomato paste, and browned beef, and stir to combine. Bring the mixture to a boil over high heat and then cover the pot and reduce the heat to low. Simmer for 45 minutes, stirring occasionally. Stir in the carrots and the remaining ¼ teaspoon of salt and ⅛ teaspoon of pepper. Bring the mixture to a boil over high heat, and then reduce the heat to low, cover, and simmer until the vegetables have softened, about 30 minutes more.
4. *To serve:* In each of four bowls, spoon 1¾ cups of the stew. Enjoy warm.

recipe continues 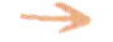

5. *To meal prep:* In each of four resealable containers, spoon 1¾ cups of the stew. Cover and refrigerate for up to 4 days or freeze for up to 2 months.
6. *To reheat:* To defrost, transfer to the refrigerator overnight. To reheat, transfer to a microwave-safe plate and microwave on high for 2 minutes. Let stand for 2 minutes to allow the heat to distribute evenly.

Nutrition Information (per serving): Calories 300; Total Fat 15g; Saturated Fat 3g; Protein 32g; Total Carbohydrates 14g; Fiber 3g; Total Sugars 5g (Includes Added Sugars 0g); Sodium 620mg

Toby's Tip: This is a perfect dish to make a double or triple batch of and freeze for a cold day.

One-Pot Creamy Orzo *with* Pork, Mushrooms, and Spinach

As a single working mom of three kids, one-pot meals saved my sanity. This creamy one-pot orzo is made with very lean pork tenderloin and just enough milk, butter, and Parmesan cheese to add an umami flavor without overloading on saturated fat and sodium.

PREP TIME 15 min // **COOK TIME** 37 min // **TOTAL TIME** 52 min // **SERVINGS** 4 // **SERVING SIZE** 1¼ cups

Meal Prep, Freezer-Friendly, One Pot/Pan

- 1 pound pork tenderloin, cut into 1-inch rounds
- ½ teaspoon kosher salt, divided
- ¼ teaspoon ground black pepper, divided
- 3 tablespoons olive oil, divided
- 1 medium yellow onion, chopped
- 2 cloves garlic, minced
- 8 ounces cremini or baby bella mushrooms, sliced
- 1 cup dried orzo
- 1¾ cups low-sodium chicken broth or water
- 1 teaspoon ground paprika
- 1 teaspoon dried thyme
- ⅛ teaspoon red pepper flakes
- 3 cups loosely packed baby spinach leaves
- 3 tablespoons ultra-filtered reduced-fat (2 percent) milk
- 1 tablespoon unsalted butter
- ¼ cup Parmesan cheese, shredded

1. Sprinkle the pork rounds with ¼ teaspoon of the salt and ⅛ teaspoon of the pepper.
2. Heat 2 tablespoons of the oil in a large sauté pan over medium heat. Once the oil is shimmering, add the pork tenderloin and cook until browned on both sides, about 8 minutes. Transfer the pork rounds to a clean plate; set aside.
3. Heat the remaining 1 tablespoon of oil in the same sauté pan over medium heat. Once the oil is shimmering, add the onion and garlic, and cook until the onion is translucent and garlic is fragrant, about 3 minutes. Add the mushrooms and cook until softened, about 8 minutes. Add the orzo, broth or water, paprika, thyme, red pepper flakes, and remaining ¼ teaspoon salt and ⅛ teaspoon pepper; stir to combine. Increase the heat to high and bring mixture to a boil and then reduce the heat to medium-low and cook, covered, until the orzo is tender, about 10 minutes. Add the pork and stir to combine. Continue cooking, uncovered, for 5 minutes. Add the spinach and cook until wilted, about 3 minutes.
4. Remove the pan from the heat and stir in the milk, butter, and cheese until creamy.
5. *To serve:* On each of four plates, spoon 1¼ cups of the orzo; enjoy warm.

recipe continues 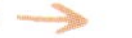

6. *To meal prep:* In each of four resealable containers, spoon 1¼ cups of the orzo. Cover and refrigerate for up to 4 days or freeze for up to 2 months.
7. *To reheat:* To defrost, transfer to the refrigerator overnight. To reheat, transfer to a microwave-safe plate and microwave on high for 1½ minutes. Let stand for 2 minutes to allow the heat to distribute evenly.

Nutrition Information (per serving): Calories 469; Total Fat 19g; Saturated Fat 5g; Protein 34g; Total Carbohydrates 40g; Fiber 4g; Total Sugars 3g (Includes Added Sugars 0g); Sodium 573mg

Toby's Tip: Swap the pork tenderloin for turkey or chicken breast tenderloin.

Pork Adobo over Rice

This version of the classic Filipino dish balances salty soy sauce with sour vinegar and a variety of aromatics. The pork chunks are slow-cooked in this unbelievable sauce until they become so tender that they fall apart.

PREP TIME 15 min // **COOK TIME** 1 hour, 31 min // **TOTAL TIME** 1 hour, 46 min // **SERVINGS** 4

SERVING SIZE ¾ cup pork + ¾ cup rice

Meal Prep, Freezer-Friendly | **Dairy-free**

FOR THE PORK

1½ pounds boneless pork shoulder, picnic or butt, cut into 2-inch pieces

¼ teaspoon kosher salt

¼ teaspoon ground black pepper, divided

2 tablespoons olive oil

5 cloves garlic, minced

1½ cups low-sodium beef broth or water

¼ cup reduced-sodium soy sauce

¼ cup apple cider vinegar

4 bay leaves

FOR THE RICE

2 cups water

1 cup dry Jasmine rice

1. Sprinkle the pork pieces with salt and ⅛ teaspoon of the pepper.
2. Heat the oil in a large pot over medium heat. Once the oil is shimmering, add the garlic and cook until fragrant, about 1 minute. Add the pork, broth or water, soy sauce, vinegar, bay leaf, and the remaining ⅛ teaspoon of pepper, and bring the mixture to a boil over high heat. Cover, reduce the heat to low, and simmer the beef until tender, about 1 hour, turning the meat over occasionally.
3. Remove cover and continue cooking on low, until the liquid is reduced by at least half, an additional 20 to 30 minutes. Discard bay leaf before serving.
4. In a medium saucepan, bring the water and rice to a boil over high heat. Reduce the heat to medium-low, cover, and simmer until the rice is tender, about 15 minutes.
5. *To serve:* On each of four plates, spoon ¾ cup of rice and top with ¾ cup of the adobo pork.
6. *To meal prep:* In each of four resealable containers, spoon ¾ cup of rice next to ¾ cup of the adobo. Cover and refrigerate for up to 4 days.

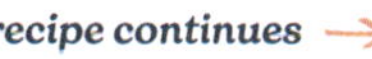
recipe continues →

7. *To reheat:* Transfer to a microwave-safe plate and microwave on high for 2 minutes. Let it stand for 2 minutes to allow the heat to distribute evenly.

Nutrition Information (per serving): Calories 447; Total Fat 13g; Saturated Fat 3g; Protein 39g; Total Carbohydrates 40g; Fiber 0g; Total Sugars 1g (Includes Added Sugars 0g); Sodium 680mg

Toby's Tip: Pork shoulder picnic is leaner compared to the pork shoulder butt. However, because the pork shoulder butt has more marbling (or fat) it will come out more tender and moist.

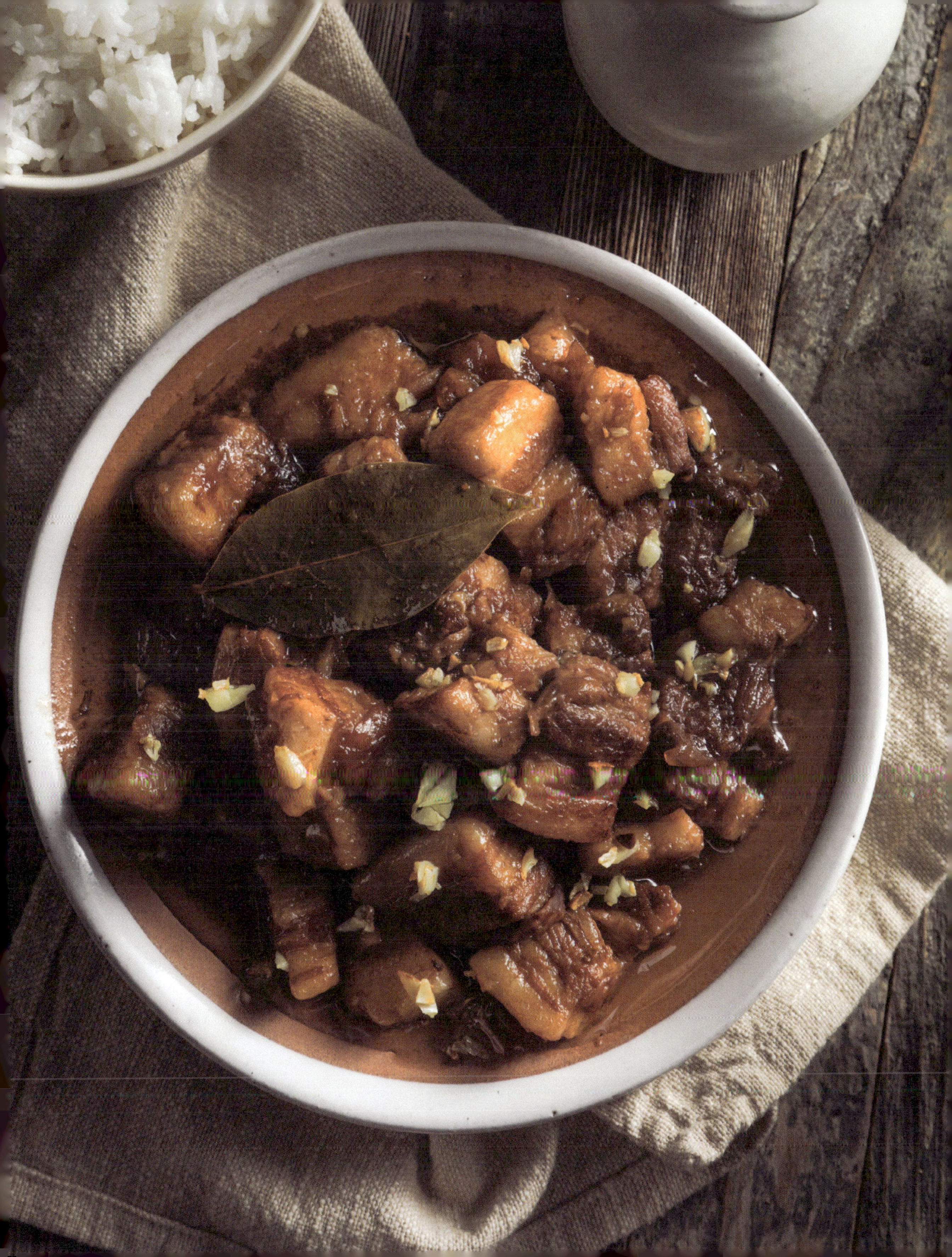

Pomegranate-Glazed Pork Chops *with* Brussels Sprouts

Don't settle for bland pork chops! This delicious pomegranate glaze transforms the lean cut of meat with a burst of flavor and contains plenty of antioxidants besides.

PREP TIME 15 min // **COOK TIME** 50 min // **TOTAL TIME** 1 hour, 5 min // **SERVINGS** 4

SERVING SIZE 1 pork chop + 2 tablespoons glaze + ½ cup Brussels sprouts

Meal Prep, Freezer-Friendly | Gluten-Free

- Nonstick cooking spray
- 1 pound Brussels sprouts, trimmed and halved
- ¼ cup olive oil, divided
- ¾ teaspoon kosher salt, divided
- 4 (5 ounce) boneless pork chops
- ⅛ teaspoon ground black pepper
- 1 shallot, chopped
- 1 cup 100 percent pomegranate juice
- 2 teaspoons liquid honey
- 1 tablespoon balsamic vinegar
- 1 teaspoon dried thyme
- 1 teaspoon dried parsley
- 1 tablespoon unsalted butter

1. Preheat the oven to 425°F. Coat a rimmed baking sheet with cooking spray.
2. In a large bowl, add the Brussels sprouts, 2 tablespoons of the oil, and ½ teaspoon of the salt. Arrange in a single layer on the prepared baking dish. Roast the Brussels sprouts until crispy and browned, 20 to 22 minutes, tossing halfway through. Set aside to slightly cool.
3. Sprinkle the pork chops with the remaining ¼ teaspoon of salt and pepper. Heat the remaining 2 tablespoons of oil in a large skillet over medium heat. Once the oil is shimmering, add the pork chops and cook until the internal temperature reaches 145°F, 4 to 6 minutes on each side. Using tongs, cook the chops on their side, about 1 minute per side. Remove the pork chops from the heat; set aside.
4. In the same hot skillet over medium heat, add the shallot and cook until softened and translucent, about 2 minutes, scraping up the brown bits from the bottom of the pan. Add the pomegranate juice, liquid honey, vinegar, thyme, and parsley, and whisk to combine. Bring the mixture to a boil over high heat and then reduce the heat to medium-low and simmer until the liquid is reduced by about one-third, about 10 minutes. Remove the skillet from the heat and whisk in the butter until smooth.

5. *To serve:* On each of four plates, place 1 pork chop and ½ cup Brussels sprouts. Drizzle pork with 2 tablespoons of the pomegranate glaze.

6. *To meal prep*: In each of four resealable containers, place 1 pork chop and ½ cup Brussels sprouts. Drizzle the pork with 2 tablespoons of the pomegranate glaze. Cover and refrigerate for up to 4 days or freeze for up to 2 months.

7. *To reheat*: To defrost, transfer to the refrigerator overnight. To reheat, transfer to a microwave-safe plate and microwave on high for 2 minutes. Let stand for 2 minutes to allow the heat to distribute evenly.

Nutrition Information (per serving): Calories 408; Total Fat 21g; Saturated Fat 5g; Protein 35g; Total Carbohydrates 23g; Fiber 5g; Total Sugars 14g (Includes Added Sugars 3g); Sodium 598mg

Toby's Tip: Serve with Farro with Mushrooms on page 259.

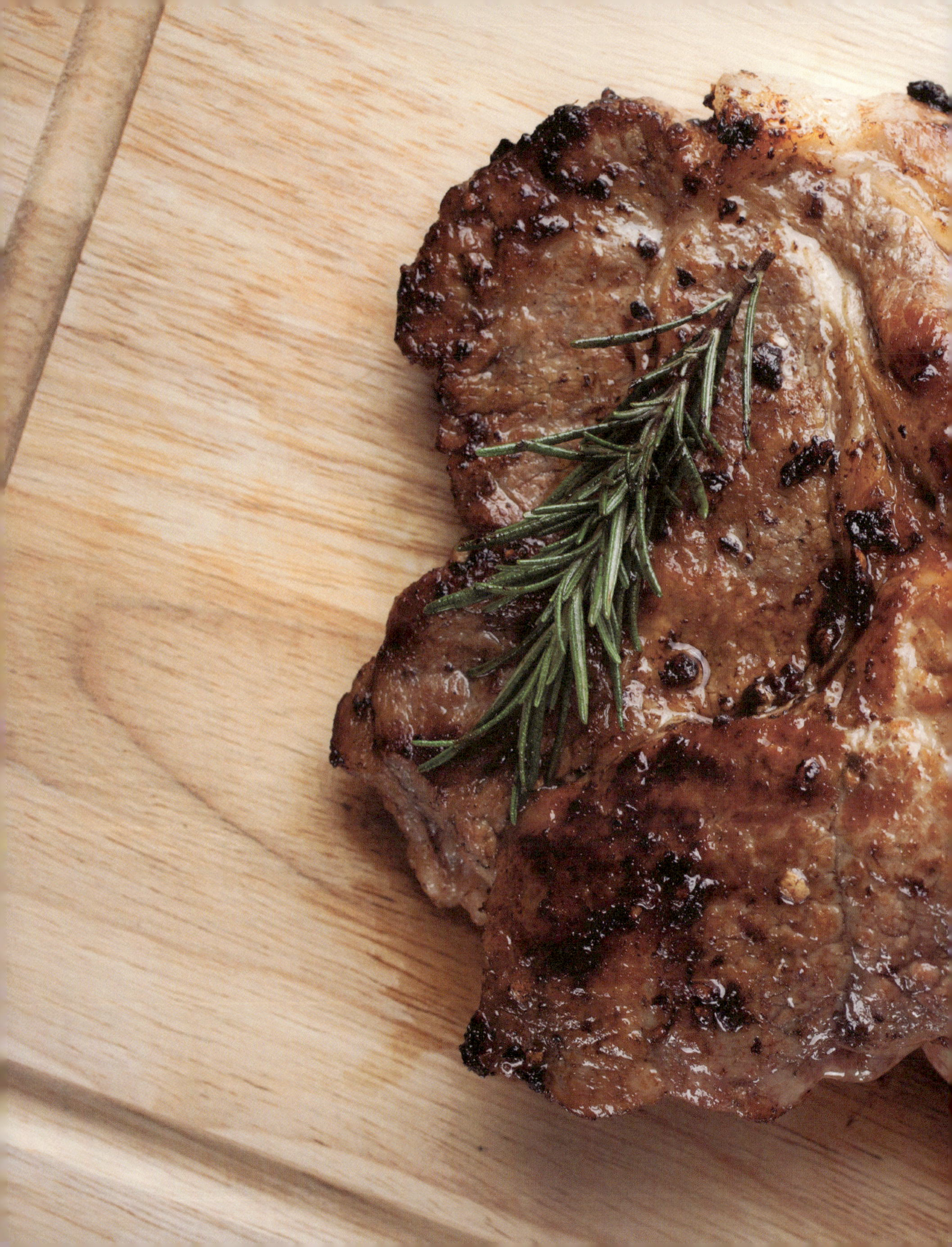

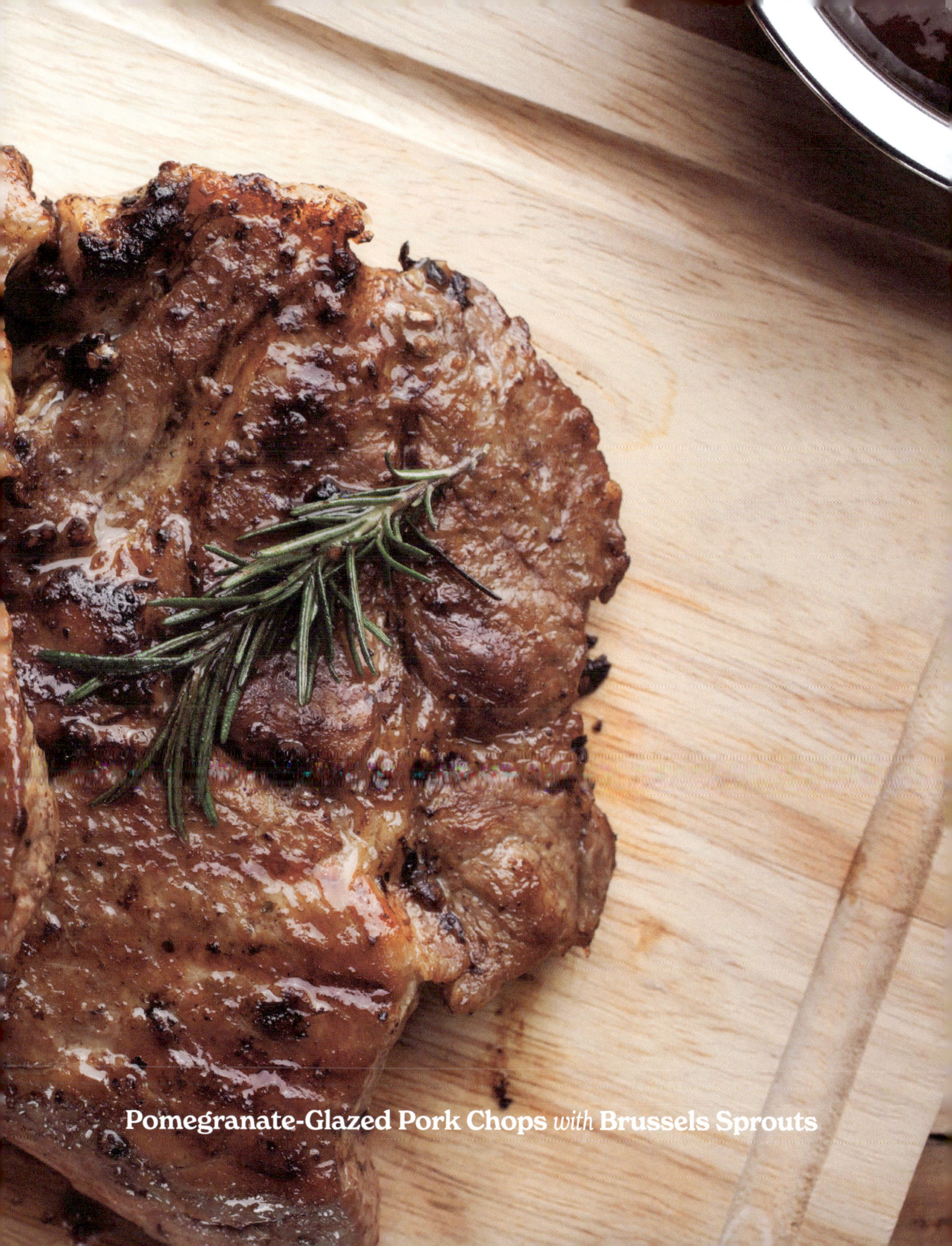

Pomegranate-Glazed Pork Chops *with* **Brussels Sprouts**

Ground Pork Stir-Fry *with* Mushroom, Zucchini, and Carrots

Swap out the classic stir-fry protein for ground meat to create a different texture and deeper flavor. It's a simple change that makes a great addition to your weekly dinner menu.

PREP TIME 20 min // **COOK TIME** 1 hour, 6 min // **TOTAL TIME** 1 hour, 26 min // **SERVINGS** 4

SERVING SIZE 1¼ cups stir-fry + ¾ cup rice

Meal Prep, Freezer-Friendly | **Dairy-free**

FOR THE RICE

2 cups water

1 cup brown basmati rice

FOR THE BROWN SAUCE

1 cup low-sodium chicken broth, divided

¼ cup reduced-sodium soy sauce

2 tablespoons unseasoned rice vinegar

1 tablespoon sesame oil

2 teaspoons liquid honey

½ teaspoon ground ginger

⅛ teaspoon ground black pepper

1 tablespoon cornstarch

FOR THE STIR-FRY

1 tablespoon olive oil

1 pound ground pork (at least 90 percent lean)

2 cloves garlic, minced

6 ounces Portobello mushrooms, cut into 2-inch pieces

1 medium zucchini, cut into 1-inch rounds

1 medium carrot, shredded

1. *For the rice:* In a medium saucepan, bring the water and rice to a boil over high heat. Cover and reduce the heat to medium-low. Simmer until the rice is tender, about 30 minutes. Fluff with a fork and set aside.
2. *For the brown sauce:* In a medium skillet, whisk together ¾ cup of the broth and the soy sauce, vinegar, sesame oil, liquid honey, ginger, and black pepper. Bring the mixture to a boil over high heat. Reduce the heat and simmer, whisking occasionally, until about one-third of the liquid is reduced, 10 to 12 minutes.
3. Meanwhile, in a small bowl, whisk together the remaining ¼ cup of broth and cornstarch until the mixture is slightly thickened, about 1 minute.
4. Whisk the cornstarch mixture into the brown sauce, and cook until the mixture has thickened, 4 to 5 minutes. Set aside to slightly cool.

5. *For the stir-fry:* Heat the oil in a large wok over high heat. Add the pork and cook, breaking up the chunks with the back of the spoon, until browned on all sides and the pork reaches an internal temperature of 145°F, about 8 minutes. Transfer the pork to a clean plate.
6. In the same wok with the remaining oil inside, cook the garlic over medium-high heat until fragrant, about 1 minute. Add the mushrooms and zucchini, and cook, stirring occasionally, until the vegetables have slightly softened, about 5 minutes. Add the carrots and cook, stirring occasionally, until slightly softened, about 3 minutes. Add the pork and toss to combine, about 1 minute. Add the sauce and toss to evenly coat, 1 minute.
7. *To serve:* On each of four plates, spoon ¾ cup of the rice and top with 1¼ cups of the stir-fry.
8. *To meal prep:* In each of four resealable containers, spoon ¾ cups of the rice and 1¼ cups of the stir-fry. Cover and refrigerate for up to 4 days or freeze for up to 2 months.
9. *To reheat:* To defrost, transfer to the refrigerator overnight or up to 4 days. To reheat, transfer to a small saucepan and bring the sauce to a boil over high heat, and then reduce the heat and cook until heated through, about 5 minutes. Alternatively, transfer the stir-fry and rice to a microwave-safe plate and microwave on high for 1½ minutes. Let stand for 2 minutes to allow the heat to evenly distribute.

Nutrition Information (per serving): Calories 490; Total Fat 20g; Saturated Fat 5g; Protein 29g; Total Carbohydrates 50g; Fiber 3g; Total Sugars 8g (Includes Added Sugars 3g); Sodium 542mg

Toby's Tip: Swap in ground turkey, chicken, or lamb for ground pork. Turkey and chicken should be cooked to a minimum internal temperature of 165°F.

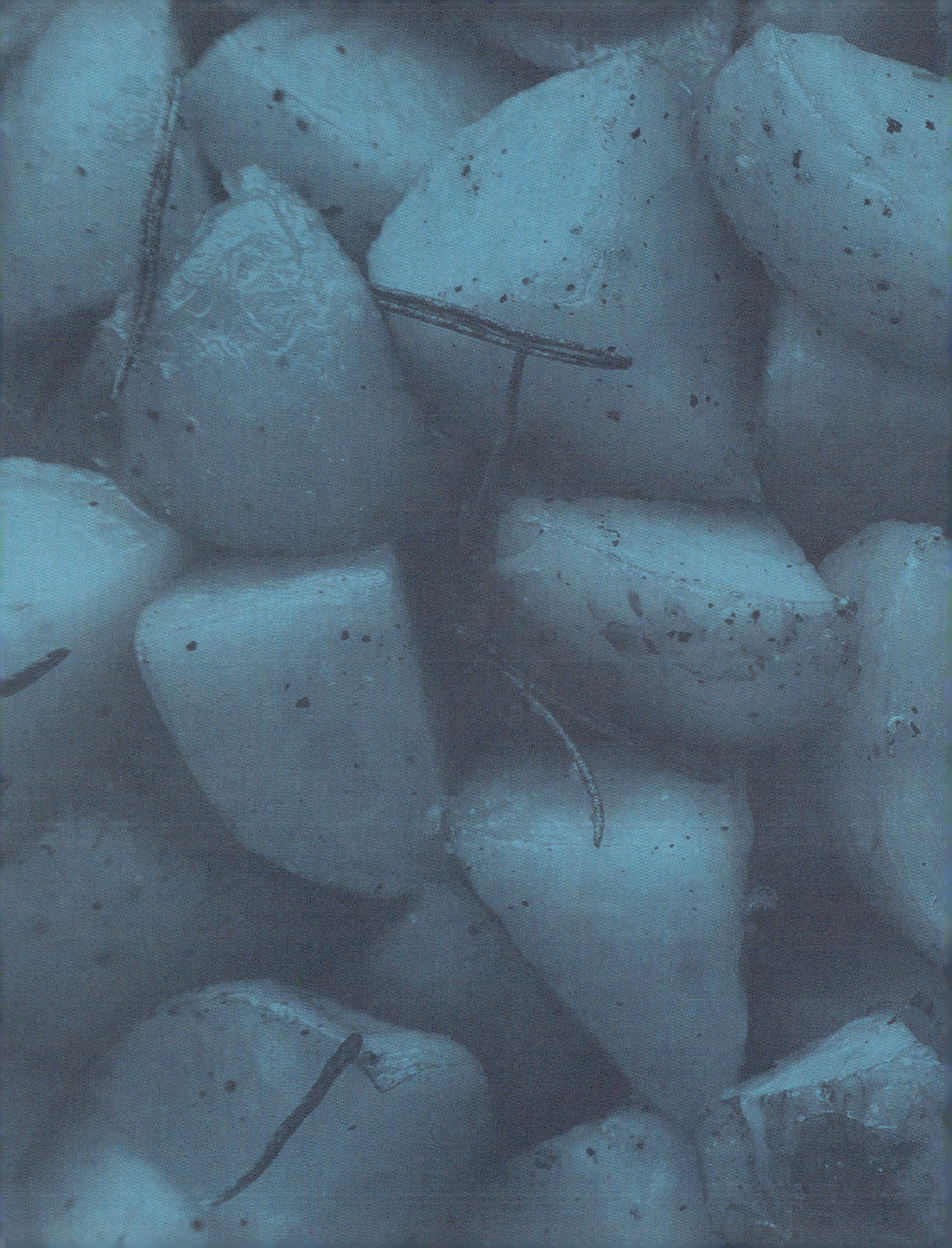

CHAPTER 10

Side Dishes

Everyday Side Salad *with* Red Wine Vinaigrette

This staple salad can be added to pretty much any meal. It helps balance your plate with vitamins and minerals, which assist protein in doing its job.

PREP TIME 20 min // **COOK TIME** 0 min // **TOTAL TIME** 20 min // **SERVINGS** 4

SERVING SIZE 2 cups salad + 2 tablespoons dressing

Meal Prep, 30 Minutes or Less | Vegetarian, Gluten-Free, Dairy-Free

FOR THE SALAD

6 cups loosely packed romaine lettuce, chopped

1 plum tomato, thinly sliced lengthwise and then cut into ½-inch slices

1 Kirby or mini cucumber, sliced lengthwise and cut into ¾-inch half-moons

1 medium carrot, shredded

FOR THE RED WINE VINAIGRETTE

¼ cup red wine vinegar

2 teaspoons Dijon mustard

1 teaspoon liquid honey

½ teaspoon ground oregano

¼ teaspoon kosher salt

⅛ teaspoon garlic powder

⅓ cup extra-virgin olive oil

1. In a large salad bowl, add the lettuce and top with tomatoes, cucumber, and carrots.
2. *For the vinaigrette:* In a small bowl, whisk together the red wine vinegar, Dijon, honey, oregano, salt, and garlic powder. While continually whisking, slowly drizzle in the oil until fully incorporated.
3. Drizzle the dressing over the salad and toss to combine.
4. *To meal prep*: In four resealable containers, place 2 cups of the salad. In four smaller containers, spoon 2 tablespoons of the dressing. Cover containers and refrigerate for up to 4 days. Dress the salad before serving.

Nutrition Information (per serving): Calories 195; Total Fat 19g; Saturated Fat 3g; Protein 1g; Total Carbohydrates 7g; Fiber 2g; Total Sugars 4g (Includes Added Sugars 1.5g); Sodium 160mg

Toby's Tip: If you don't want to make your own dressing, opt for a lighter bottled vinaigrette made with healthy fats and stick with a 2 tablespoon max portion.

White Bean, Kale, and Cranberry Salad

This side salad adds about 8 grams of protein to any main dish. It combines protein- and fiber-rich beans with healthy-fat, protein-packed nuts and is finished with a light balsamic vinaigrette.

PREP TIME 15 min // **COOK TIME** 0 min // **TOTAL TIME** 15 min // **SERVINGS** 4 // **SERVING SIZE** 1 cup

Meal Prep, 30 Minutes or Less | Vegetarian, Gluten-Free, Dairy-Free

FOR THE SALAD

3 cups loosely packed kale, chopped, thick stems removed

2 teaspoons extra-virgin olive oil

⅛ teaspoon kosher salt

1 (14.5-ounce) can low-sodium cannellini beans, rinsed and drained

¼ medium red onion, chopped

¼ cup unsweetened dried cranberries

FOR THE BALSAMIC DRESSING

2 tablespoons balsamic vinegar

1 teaspoon Dijon mustard

1 teaspoon liquid honey

⅛ teaspoon kosher salt

⅛ teaspoon ground black pepper

3 tablespoons extra-virgin olive oil

2 tablespoons chopped unsalted dry-roasted cashews

1. Place the kale in a large bowl and drizzle with the oil and salt. Using your hands, massage the kale until it starts to soften, about 5 minutes. Add the beans, onions, and cranberries. Toss to combine.
2. *For the dressing:* In a small bowl, whisk together the vinegar, mustard, honey, salt, and pepper. While continuously whisking, gradually drizzle in the oil until incorporated.
3. Drizzle the dressing on the salad and toss to evenly coat. Top with cashews.
4. *To serve:* On each of four plates, spoon 1 cup of the salad.
5. *To meal prep:* In four resealable containers, place 1 cup of the dressed salad. Cover all the containers and refrigerate for up to 4 days.

Nutrition Information (per serving): Calories 277; Total Fat 16g; Saturated Fat 2g; Protein 8g; Total Carbohydrates 28g; Fiber 6g; Total Sugars 10g (Includes Added Sugars 7g); Sodium 162mg

Toby's Tip: Swap the cannellini beans for Great Northern, adzuki, or pinto beans.

Cauliflower Gratin

Who doesn't love cheesy goodness added to their veggies? Not only does cheese add some protein, but it also adds calcium and that ooey-gooey goodness.

PREP TIME 15 min // **COOK TIME** 33 min // **TOTAL TIME** 48 min // **SERVINGS** 6 // **SERVING SIZE** 1 cup

Meal Prep, Freezer-Friendly | **Vegetarian, Gluten-Free**

- Cooking spray
- 2 heads cauliflower, roughly chopped
- 3 tablespoons olive oil
- ½ teaspoon kosher salt, divided
- ¼ teaspoon freshly ground black pepper, divided
- Nonstick cooking spray
- ⅔ cup ultra-filtered skim milk (13 grams protein per cup)
- 2 tablespoons unsalted butter, softened
- ½ teaspoon garlic powder
- 1½ cups reduced-fat shredded Mexican cheese blend

1. Preheat oven to 450°F. Coat two rimmed baking sheets with cooking spray.
2. In a large bowl, add the chopped cauliflower, oil, ¼ teaspoon salt, and ⅛ teaspoon pepper and toss to evenly coat. Divide the chopped cauliflower in half and arrange in a single layer on each of the prepared baking sheets. Roast in the preheated oven until slightly browned, 20 to 25 minutes, tossing halfway through. Remove the pans from the oven and allow to cool for 10 minutes. Reduce the oven temperature to 375°F.
3. Coat an 8 × 8-inch baking dish with nonstick cooking spray.
4. In a large bowl, using a potato masher, mash the cauliflower. Add the milk, butter, garlic powder, and the remaining ¼ teaspoon of the salt and ⅛ teaspoon of the pepper. Mix to combine.
5. Place the cauliflower mixture into the prepared baking dish. Evenly sprinkle the cheese over top and bake in the oven until the top is bubbling and slightly browned, about 8 minutes. Carefully remove the dish from the oven and allow to slightly cool, about 10 minutes.
6. *To serve:* On each of six plates, spoon 1 cup of the gratin. Serve warm.
7. *To meal prep:* In each of six resealable containers, spoon 1 cup of the gratin. Cover and refrigerate for up to 4 days or freeze for up to 2 months.

8. *To reheat:* To defrost, transfer to the refrigerator overnight. To reheat, transfer to a microwave-safe bowl and reheat on high for 1 minute; let stand 2 minutes to allow the heat to distribute evenly.

Nutrition Information (per serving): Calories 208; Total Fat 14g; Saturated Fat 6g; Protein 11g; Total Carbohydrates 11g; Fiber 4g; Total Sugars 5g (Includes Added Sugars 0g); Sodium 526mg

Toby's Tip: Enjoy as a side to the Herbed Butter Steak on page 224 (instead of Broccoli Mashed Potatoes).

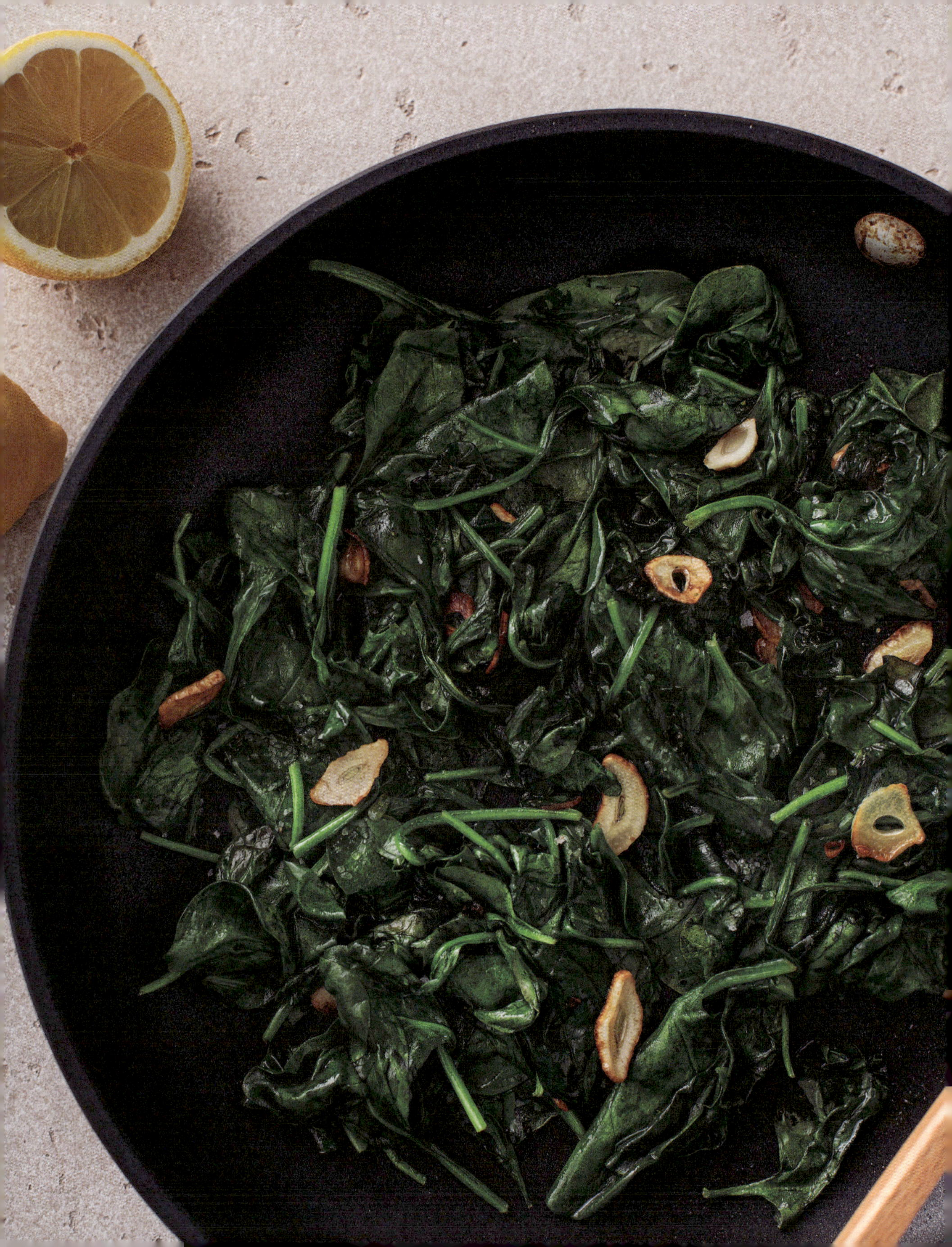

Lemon-Garlic Spinach

Sautéed spinach is a beloved and easy-to-make side that goes well with fish, chicken, and meat dishes.

PREP TIME 10 min // **COOK TIME** 4 min // **TOTAL TIME** 14 min // **SERVINGS** 4 // **SERVING SIZE** ½ cup

Meal Prep, Freezer-Friendly, One Pot/Pan, 30 Minutes or Less | Vegan, Vegetarian, Gluten-Free, Dairy-Free

2 tablespoons olive oil

4 cloves garlic, minced

1 pound loosely packed baby spinach leaves or 1½ heads spinach, trimmed and roughly chopped

Juice and zest of 1 lemon

¼ teaspoon kosher salt

⅛ teaspoon black pepper

1. Heat the oil in a medium sauté pan over medium heat. Once the oil is shimmering, add the garlic and cook until fragrant, about 30 seconds. Add about one-third of the spinach and stir until it begins to wilt, 2 to 3 minutes. Repeat with the remaining spinach until all of the spinach is wilted.
2. Remove the pan from the heat, and add the lemon juice, lemon zest, salt, and pepper; stir to combine. Serve warm.

Nutrition Information (per serving): Calories 93; Total Fat 7g; Saturated Fat 1g; Protein 3g; Total Carbohydrates 6g; Fiber 3g; Total Sugars 0g (Includes Added Sugars 0g); Sodium 165mg

Toby's Tip: If you purchase bagged baby spinach that is triple washed or pre-washed, there is no need to rewash it. There is a higher chance of you contaminating it if you do.

Side Dishes

Warm Three-Bean Salad *with* Cilantro-Lime Dressing

Beans certainly have protein, but they also provide plenty of fiber, which helps promote digestion. As an added value, beans also act as prebiotics, which means that they feed beneficial gut bacteria, fostering a healthy microbiome. This, in turn, can enhance a variety of metabolic functions such as digestion, nutrient absorption, and immune function. In this bean-centric salad, you'll find a medley of beans and textures to excite your taste buds.

PREP TIME 15 min // **COOK TIME** 10 min // **TOTAL TIME** 25 min // **SERVINGS** 4 // **SERVING SIZE** ¾ cup

Meal Prep, 30 Minutes or Less | Vegan, Vegetarian, Gluten-Free, Dairy-Free

1 cup frozen shelled edamame

5 tablespoons olive oil, divided

4 ounces green beans, trimmed and cut into ½-inch pieces

1 (15.5-ounce) can low-sodium pinto beans, rinsed and drained

Juice of 1 lime

2 tablespoons fresh cilantro leaves, chopped

½ teaspoon ground cumin

¼ teaspoon garlic powder

¼ teaspoon kosher salt

⅛ teaspoon ground black pepper

1. Fill a small saucepan halfway with water and bring to a boil over high heat. Add the edamame, reduce the heat to medium-low, and cook until the edamame is tender, about 5 minutes. Drain and set aside.
2. In a medium skillet, heat 1 tablespoon of the oil over medium heat. Once the oil is shimmering, add the cooked edamame, green beans, and cannellini beans, and cook, stirring occasionally, until warmed through, about 5 minutes. Remove the skillet from the heat and set aside to slightly cool, about 10 minutes.
3. In a medium bowl, whisk together the remaining 4 tablespoons of oil, lime juice, cilantro, ground cumin, garlic powder, salt, and pepper. Transfer the bean mixture to the bowl and toss to evenly coat.
4. *To serve:* On each of four plates, spoon ¾ cup of the bean mixture. Enjoy warm or cold.
5. *To meal prep*: In each of four resealable containers, spoon ¾ cup of the bean mixture. Cover and refrigerate for up to 4 days.

6. *To reheat*: Enjoy cold or transfer to a microwave-safe bowl and microwave on high for 45 seconds; let stand 2 minutes to allow the heat to distribute evenly.

Nutrition Information (per serving): Calories 297; Total Fat 19g; Saturated Fat 3g; Protein 9g; Total Carbohydrates 23g; Fiber 7g; Total Sugars 3g (Includes Added Sugars 0g); Sodium 322mg

Toby's Tip: Serve with the Broccoli, Cauliflower, and Farro Casserole on page 175.

Roasted Vegetables

One of my go-to ways to balance the protein and carbs on my plate is to roast whatever vegetables I have on hand. Oftentimes it is broccoli, peppers, and carrots, but you can use whichever veggies you love or that are just hanging out in your refrigerator.

PREP TIME 15 min // **COOK TIME** 25 min // **TOTAL TIME** 40 min // **SERVINGS** 4 // **SERVING SIZE** 1 cup

Meal Prep, One Pot/Pan | Vegan, Vegetarian, Gluten-Free, Dairy-Free

Nonstick cooking spray

2 tablespoons extra-virgin olive oil

1 tablespoon ground flaxseed

1 teaspoon ground rosemary

¼ teaspoon kosher salt

¼ teaspoon ground black pepper

5 cups broccoli florets

2 red peppers, seeds and ribs removed, cut into 2-inch strips

4 carrots, peeled and cut into 1½ inch rounds

1. Preheat the oven to 425°F. Coat a rimmed baking sheet with nonstick cooking spray.
2. In a large bowl, whisk together the oil, ground flaxseed, rosemary, salt, and pepper. Add the broccoli, peppers, and carrots, and toss to evenly coat.
3. Transfer the vegetables to the prepared baking sheet and bake in the preheated oven for 20 to 25 minutes, turning the vegetables halfway through. Remove the baking sheet from the oven and allow to cool for 10 minutes.
4. *To serve:* On each of four plates, spoon 1 cup of the vegetables. Serve warm.
5. *To meal prep:* In each of four resealable containers, spoon 1 cup of the vegetables. Cover and refrigerate for up to 4 days.
6. *To reheat*: Transfer to a microwave-safe plate and microwave on high for 1 minute; let stand for 2 minutes to allow the heat to distribute evenly.

Nutrition Information (per serving): Calories 122; Total Fat 6g; Saturated Fat 1g; Protein 4g; Total Carbohydrates 15g; Fiber 3g; Total Sugars 5g (Includes Added Sugars 0g); Sodium 127mg

Toby's Tip: Heartier vegetables like potatoes can take longer to cook. To cut cook time, cut them into smaller pieces so they are ready quicker.

Couscous *with* Chickpeas, Peas, and Carrots

Couscous is made with semolina flour that is rolled into small balls. It is sold in tiny granules or as pearled couscous, which are larger spheres. It's a versatile ingredient that can be used as a side dish or in salads and stews.

PREP TIME 10 min // **COOK TIME** 15 min // **TOTAL TIME** 25 min // **SERVINGS** 6 // **SERVING SIZE** About ¾ cup

Meal Prep, One Pot/Pan, 30 Minutes or Less | **Vegan, Vegetarian, Dairy-Free**

1 tablespoon olive or avocado oil

1 small onion, chopped

1 clove garlic, minced

2 cups low-sodium vegetable broth or water

1 cup low-sodium chickpeas, rinsed and drained

1 cup frozen peas and carrots

1 cup dried couscous

1 teaspoon ground cumin

1 teaspoon dried thyme

¼ teaspoon kosher salt

⅛ teaspoon ground black pepper

2 tablespoons pine nuts

1. Heat the oil in a medium saucepan over medium heat. Once the oil is shimmering, add the onion and garlic, and cook until the onion has softened and garlic is fragrant, about 3 minutes. Add the broth or water, chickpeas, peas and carrots, couscous, cumin, thyme, salt, and pepper; stir to combine. Increase the heat to high and bring to a boil, and then reduce the heat to medium-low, cover, and simmer until the water is absorbed and the couscous in fluffy, about 15 minutes. Garnish with the pine nuts.
2. *To serve:* On each of six plates, spoon ¾ cup of the couscous.
3. *To meal prep:* In each of six resealable containers, spoon ¾ cup of the couscous. Cover and refrigerate for up to 4 days.
4. *To reheat:* Transfer to a microwave-safe plate and microwave on high for 1 minute; let stand for 2 minutes to allow the heat to distribute evenly.

Nutrition Information (per serving): Calories 210; Total Fat 5g; Saturated Fat 1g; Protein 7g; Total Carbohydrates 33g; Fiber 5g; Total Sugars 2g (Includes Added Sugars 0g); Sodium 167mg

Toby's Tip: Swap the chickpeas for cannellini or pinto beans.

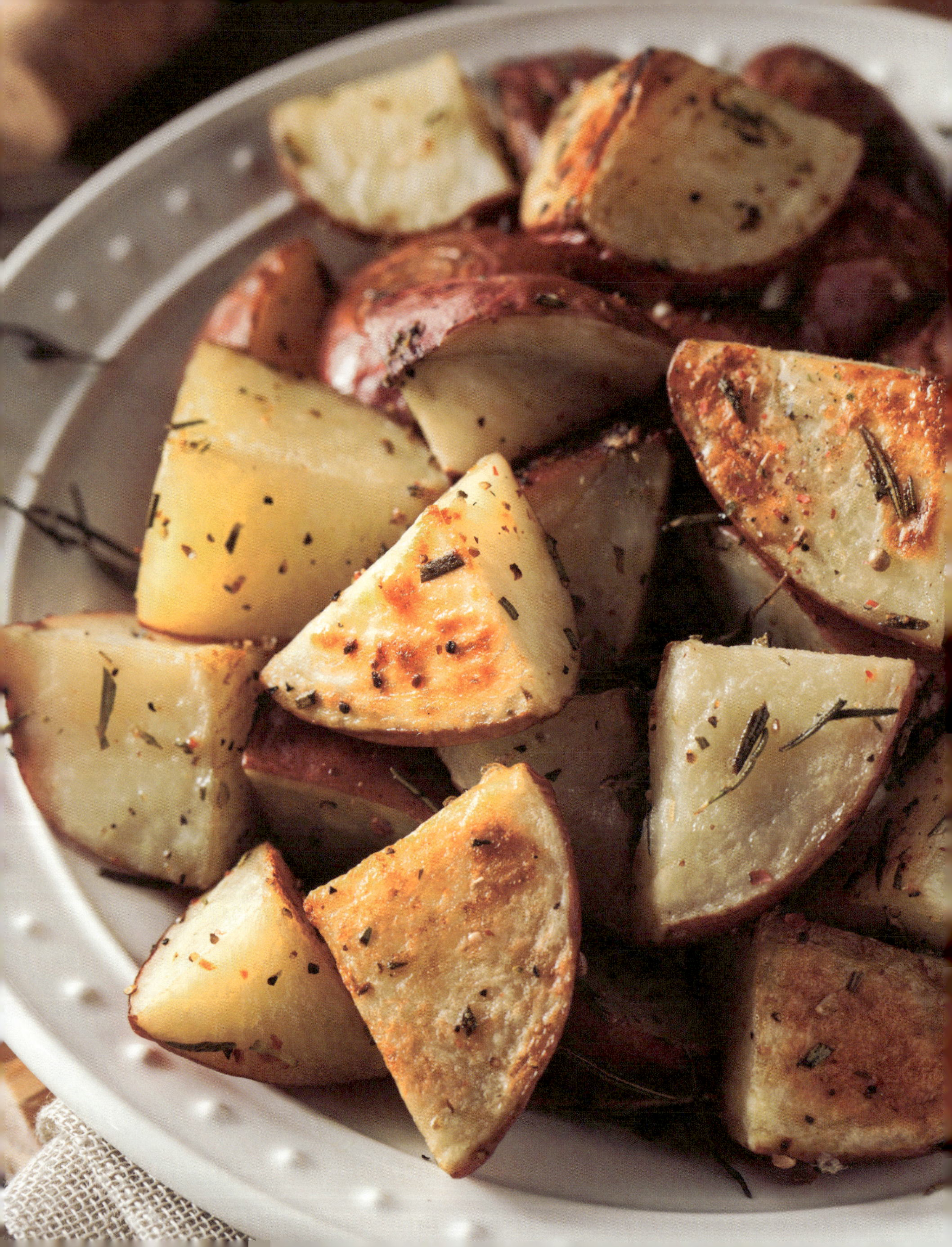

Tajín Baked Red Potatoes

Tajín is a popular Mexican seasoning made from a combination of mild chili peppers, sea salt, and dehydrated lime juice. It provides a unique balance of sweet, salty, and slight heat.

PREP TIME 15 min // **COOK TIME** 25 min // **TOTAL TIME** 40 min // **SERVINGS** 4 // **SERVING SIZE** 1 cup

Meal Prep, One Pot/Pan, 30 Minutes or Less | Vegan, Vegetarian, Gluten-Free, Dairy-Free

- 1½ pounds (4 medium) red potatoes with skin, quartered and cut into ¾-inch slices
- 2 tablespoons extra-virgin olive oil
- 2 teaspoons Tajín seasoning
- 1 teaspoon dried rosemary

1. Preheat the oven to 425°F. Line a rimmed baking sheet with parchment paper.
2. In a large bowl, drizzle the potatoes with the oil, and then sprinkle with the Tajín and dried rosemary; toss to evenly coat. Arrange the potatoes in a single layer on the prepared baking sheet.
3. Roast in the preheated oven until the potatoes are slightly browned, tossing halfway through, about 25 minutes.
4. *To serve:* On each of four plates, spoon 1 cup of the potatoes. Enjoy warm.
5. *To meal prep:* In each of four resealable containers, spoon 1 cup of the potatoes. Cover and refrigerate for up to 4 days.
6. *To reheat:* Transfer to a microwave-safe plate and microwave on high for 1½ minutes. Let stand for 2 minutes to allow the heat to distribute evenly.

Nutrition Information (per serving): Calories 179; Total Fat 7g; Saturated Fat 1g; Protein 3g; Total Carbohydrates 27g; Fiber 3g; Total Sugars 2g (Includes Added Sugars 0g); Sodium 411mg

Toby's Tip: For a simple change in this recipe, swap the Tajín for Italian seasoning and ¼ teaspoon salt.

Quinoa *with* Cucumber, Tomatoes, and Mozzarella

This fresh and flavorful side features protein-packed quinoa, crisp cucumbers, juicy tomatoes, and creamy mozzarella cheese. It's a side dish that can balance any protein with carbs and veggies.

PREP TIME 45 min // **COOK TIME** 15 min // **TOTAL TIME** 1 hour // **SERVINGS** 8 // **SERVING SIZE** ⅔ cup

Meal Prep | **Vegetarian, Gluten-Free**

1 cup dry quinoa

3 cups water

2 tablespoons extra-virgin olive oil

Juice of 1 lemon

2 teaspoons dried parsley

½ teaspoon kosher salt

¼ teaspoon ground black pepper

2 Kirby or mini cucumbers, chopped

1 medium red bell pepper, seeds and ribs removed, chopped

2 plum tomatoes, chopped

½ cup (about 3 ounces) mozzarella pearls

1. In a medium saucepan, add the quinoa and water and bring to a boil over high heat. Reduce the heat to medium-low, cover, and simmer until fluffy, about 15 minutes. Drain any excess water and allow to cool for 10 minutes.
2. In a large bowl, whisk together the oil, lemon juice, parsley, salt, and pepper. Add the cooled quinoa, cucumbers, bell pepper, and tomatoes; toss to evenly coat. Add the cheese and toss to combine. Cover and refrigerate for 30 minutes or up to 4 days to allow the flavors to meld. Serve cold.
3. *To serve*: On each of four plates, spoon ⅔ cup of the quinoa.
4. *To meal prep:* In each of four resealable containers, spoon ⅔ cup of the quinoa. Cover and refrigerate for up to 4 days. Enjoy cold.

Nutrition Information (per serving): Calories 200; Total Fat 10g; Saturated Fat 3g; Protein 7g; Total Carbohydrates 21g; Fiber 3g; Total Sugars 2g (Includes Added Sugars 0g); Sodium 119mg

Toby's Tip: Swap the quinoa for farro, couscous, or orzo.

Farro *with* Mushrooms

Farro is a nutty-flavored, chewy whole-wheat "ancient grain." It's packed with fiber and protein, and contains iron, magnesium, and B vitamins. One of my favorite ways to enjoy it is with mushrooms, which add a nice umami flavor to the nuttiness of the farro.

PREP TIME 15 min // **COOK TIME** 49 min // **TOTAL TIME** 1 hour, 4 min // **SERVINGS** 4 // **SERVING SIZE** 1 cup

Meal Prep, One Pot/Pan, 30 Minutes or Less | Vegan, Vegetarian, Dairy-Free

- 2 tablespoons olive or avocado oil
- 2 cloves garlic, minced
- 1 (8-ounce) container baby bella or cremini mushrooms, thinly sliced
- 1 cup dry farro
- 2 ¾ cups water
- 1 teaspoon dried parsley
- ½ teaspoon kosher salt
- ¼ teaspoon ground black pepper

1. Heat the oil in a medium saucepan over medium heat. Once the oil is shimmering, add the garlic and cook until fragrant, about 30 seconds. Add the mushrooms and cook until softened, about 8 minutes. Add the farro, water, parsley, salt, and pepper; stir to combine. Increase the heat to high and bring the mixture to a boil, and then reduce the heat to medium-low, cover, and cook until the farro is tender, about 40 minutes. Fluff with a fork.
2. *To serve:* In each of four bowls, spoon 1 cup of the farro mixture.
3. *To meal prep*: In each of four resealable bowls, spoon 1 cup of the farro, cover, and refrigerate for up to 4 days.
4. *To reheat*: Transfer the farro to a microwave-safe plate and microwave on high for 1 minute. Let sit for 2 minutes to allow the heat to distribute evenly.

Nutrition Information (per serving): Calories 167; Total Fat 6g; Saturated Fat 1g; Protein 5g; Total Carbohydrates 24g; Fiber 5g; Total Sugars 1g (Includes Added Sugars 0g); Sodium 113mg

Toby's Tip: For more flavor and a touch more protein, stir in 1 to 2 tablespoons of grated Parmesan cheese.

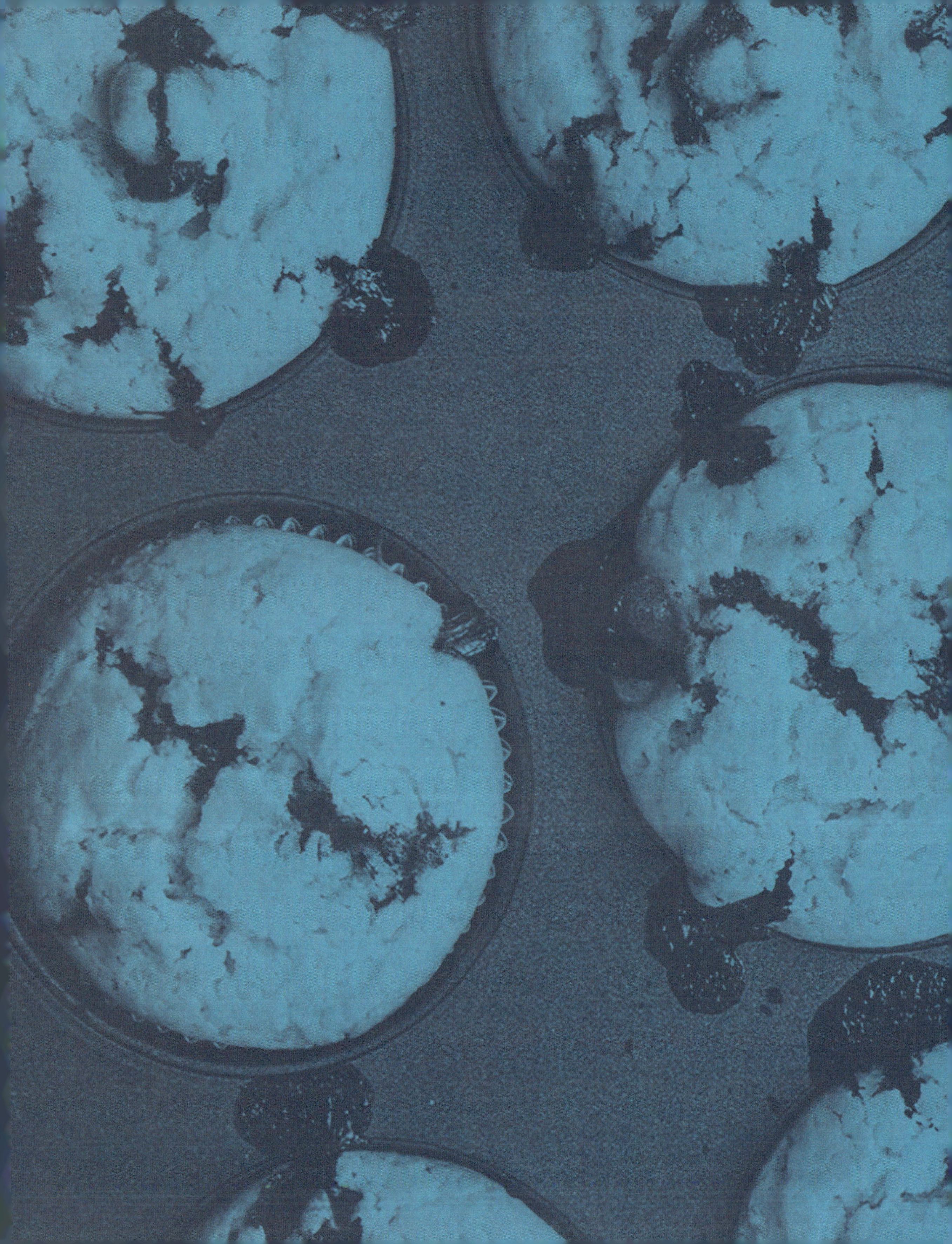

CHAPTER 11

Higher-Protein Snacks and Sweets

Protein Trail Mix

The secret of this trail mix is to combine the protein-filled nuts with a bit of sweet and tart flavors to get a whopping 9 grams of protein per serving. Snacks like this can help meet protein needs throughout the day.

PREP TIME 10 min // **COOK TIME** 0 min // **TOTAL TIME** 10 min // **SERVINGS** 6 // **SERVING SIZE** ⅓ cup

Meal Prep, One Pot/Pan, 30 Minutes or Less | Vegetarian, Gluten-Free

⅓ cup unsalted dry-roasted peanuts

⅓ cup unsalted dry-roasted pumpkin seeds

⅔ cup dry-roasted salted edamame or chickpeas

⅓ cup unsalted dry-roasted almonds

⅓ cup unsweetened dried tart cherries

¼ cup semi-sweet chocolate chips

1. In a medium bowl, add the peanuts, pumpkin seeds, edamame or chickpeas, almonds, cherries, and chocolate chips, and mix to evenly distribute.
2. *To meal prep:* In each of six resealable bags or containers, spoon ⅓ cup of the trail mix. Store in a cool, dry place for up to 2 weeks.

Nutrition Information (per serving): Calories 230; Total Fat 13g; Saturated Fat 3g; Protein 9g; Total Carbohydrates 22g; Fiber 5g; Total Sugars 13g (Includes Added Sugars 5g); Sodium 52mg

Toby's Tip: To make the trail mix vegan and dairy-free, use carob chips or dark chocolate chips with at least 60 percent cacao.

Spicy Black Bean Dip

This isn't your average dip—it's a flavor-packed, bean-based blend loaded with protein and fiber. Together with the dipping vegetables, this snack provides a whopping 8 grams of protein (that's great for a dip!), making it a perfect go-to snack option.

PREP TIME 20 min // **COOK TIME** 0 min // **TOTAL TIME** 20 min // **SERVINGS** 4

SERVING SIZE ¼ cup dip + one-quarter of the vegetables

Meal Prep, One Pot/Pan, 30 Minutes or Less | **Vegan, Vegetarian, Gluten-Free, Dairy-Free**

- 1 (14.5-ounce) can low-sodium black beans, rinsed and drained
- ½ cup (2 ounces) roasted red peppers, roughly chopped
- ½ jalapeño pepper, seeds and ribs removed, roughly chopped
- 3 tablespoons nutritional yeast
- 1½ teaspoons lime juice
- 1 clove garlic, crushed
- ½ teaspoon ground coriander seed
- ¼ teaspoon kosher salt
- ⅛ teaspoon ground black pepper
- 1 cup baby carrots
- 2 medium stalks celery, cut into 1½ inch sticks

1. In a blender or food processor, add black beans, roasted peppers, jalapeño, nutritional yeast, lime juice, garlic, coriander, salt, and pepper. Cover and blend on high speed until smooth, about 1 minute. If the mixture is too thick for your liking, add 1 tablespoon of water at a time and blend on high for 30 seconds until it reaches desired consistency.
2. *To serve:* In each of four bowls, spoon ¼ cup of dip and one-quarter of the vegetables.
3. *To meal prep:* In each of four resealable containers, spoon ¼ cup of the dip and one-quarter of the vegetables. Cover and refrigerate for up to 4 days.

Nutrition Information (per serving): Calories 127; Total Fat 1g; Saturated Fat 0g; Protein 8g; Total Carbohydrates 22g; Fiber 9g; Total Sugars 2g (Includes Added Sugars 0g); Sodium 389mg

Toby's Tip: Swap the black beans for pinto beans.

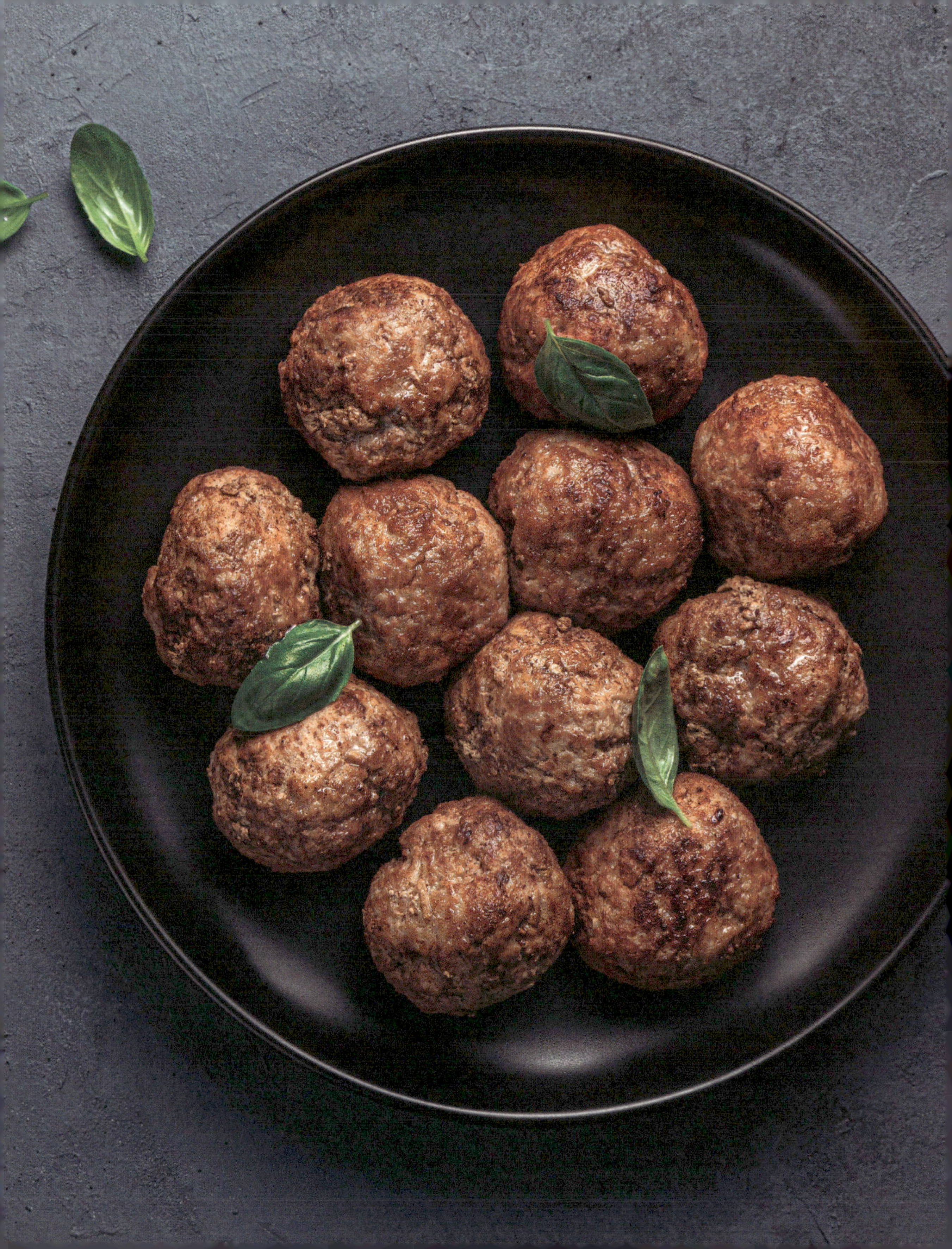

Meatballs *with* Tart Cherry Sauce

If you're craving a meat-filled snack, I've got you covered. These savory meatballs are made using lean ground meat, but a tart-yet-sweet cherry sauce transforms them into the most incredibly moist dish.

PREP TIME 30 min // **COOK TIME** 28 min // **TOTAL TIME** 58 min // **SERVINGS** 6 // **SERVING SIZE** 2 meatballs

Meal Prep, Freezer-Friendly | Dairy-free

FOR THE MEATBALLS

Nonstick cooking spray

2 teaspoons olive oil

½ small yellow onion, chopped

2 cloves garlic, minced

1 tablespoon Worcestershire sauce

1 tablespoon tomato paste

1 pound ground beef (at least 90 percent lean)

¼ cup unseasoned breadcrumbs

1 large egg, beaten

1 teaspoon Italian seasoning

1 teaspoon smoked paprika

½ teaspoon kosher salt

¼ teaspoon mustard powder

⅛ teaspoon ground black pepper

FOR THE CHERRY SAUCE

1 tablespoon olive oil

1 shallot, chopped

1 cup frozen pitted sweet dark or tart cherries

½ cup low-sodium vegetable broth

1 tablespoon balsamic vinegar

2 teaspoons liquid honey

1 teaspoon dried thyme

¼ teaspoon kosher salt

⅛ teaspoon ground black pepper

1 tablespoon unsalted butter, cut into 4 pieces

1. Preheat the oven to 350°F. Coat a rimmed baking sheet with nonstick cooking spray.
2. *To make the meatballs:* Heat the oil in a medium skillet over medium heat. Once the oil is shimmering, add the onion and garlic, and cook until the onions are soft and translucent and garlic is fragrant, about 3 minutes. Remove the skillet from the heat and allow to slightly cool, about 5 minutes.
3. Transfer the slightly cooled onions and garlic to a large bowl. Add the Worcestershire sauce and tomato paste and toss to coat the vegetables. Add the ground beef, breadcrumbs, egg, Italian seasoning, smoked paprika, salt, mustard powder, and pepper. Using clean hands, mix the ingredients until well combined.
4. Using a standard ice-cream scoop, portion one meatball and, using clean hands, roll it into a 2-inch ball. Place onto the prepared baking sheet. Repeat with the remaining mixture (you should end up with 12 meatballs).

recipe continues 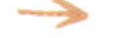

5. Place the baking sheet into the preheated oven and bake the meatballs until a thermometer inserted into the center of several meatballs reaches 155°F, 15 to 20 minutes. Remove the baking sheet from the oven and set aside for the meatballs to cool, about 15 minutes.
6. *To make the sauce:* Heat the oil in a medium saucepan over medium heat. Once the oil is shimmering, add the shallot and cook until fragrant, about 2 minutes. Add the cherries, vegetable stock, balsamic vinegar, honey, thyme, salt, and pepper; stir to combine. Increase the heat to high and bring the mixture to a boil, then reduce the heat to medium-low and simmer, stirring occasionally, until the mixture thickens and the liquid is reduced by about one-third, about 20 minutes. Using a potato masher, mash the cherries and stir to combine. Slowly stir in one piece of butter at a time until the mixture is glossy. Transfer the meatballs to the saucepan and toss to evenly coat meatballs.
7. *To serve:* On each of six plates, place 2 meatballs with sauce.
8. *To meal prep:* In each of six resealable containers, place 2 meatballs with sauce. Cover all the containers and refrigerate for up to 4 days.
9. *To reheat*: Transfer to a microwave-safe plate and microwave on high for 1 minute. Let stand for 2 minutes to allow the heat to distribute evenly.

Nutrition Information (per serving): Calories 245; Total Fat 14g; Saturated Fat 5g; Protein 17g; Total Carbohydrates 12g; Fiber 1g; Total Sugars 7g (Includes Added Sugars 2g); Sodium 228mg

Toby's Tip: Swap the ground beef with ground turkey, chicken, lamb, or pork.

Banana Walnut Protein Bread

Traditional banana bread doesn't have much protein. This version, however, is made with oats, walnuts, and a scoop of whey protein powder to give you a respectable 9 grams of protein per slice.

PREP TIME 25 min // **COOK TIME** 25 min // **TOTAL TIME** 50 min // **SERVINGS** 8 // **SERVING SIZE** 1 slice

Meal Prep, Freezer-Friendly | Vegetarian, Gluten-Free

- Cooking spray
- 2 cups + 2 tablespoons gluten-free rolled oats
- 1 (29-gram) scoop unsweetened whey protein isolate powder (25g protein per scoop)
- 2 teaspoons baking powder
- 1 teaspoon ground cinnamon
- ½ teaspoon salt
- 2 large eggs
- ¼ cup unsalted butter, softened
- ¼ cup liquid honey
- 3 tablespoons avocado or canola oil
- 1 teaspoon vanilla extract
- 3 medium ripe bananas, mashed
- ½ cup chopped walnuts

Nutrition Information (per serving): Calories 327; Total Fat 18g; Saturated Fat 6g; Protein 9g; Total Carbohydrates 35g; Fiber 4g; Total Sugars 25g (Includes Added Sugars g); Sodium 306mg

1. Preheat the oven to 350°F. Coat an 8-inch loaf pan with cooking spray.
2. In a medium bowl, mix together 2 cups of the oats and the protein powder, baking powder, cinnamon, and salt.
3. In a separate medium bowl, whisk together the beaten eggs and butter until smooth. Add the honey, oil, and vanilla, and whisk until incorporated. Add the mashed banana and whisk until incorporated.
4. Add the dry ingredients to the wet ingredients and stir just until combined. Gently fold in the walnuts.
5. Pour the mixture into the prepared pan, using a spatula to spread it into an even layer. Sprinkle the remaining 2 tablespoons of oats onto the top of the batter.
6. Bake in the preheated oven until the top is golden brown and a toothpick inserted into the center comes out clean, about 25 minutes. Remove the pan from the oven and allow to cool for 10 minutes. Then transfer the bread to a wire rack and let it cool for 10 to 15 minutes
7. *To serve:* Cut into 1-inch slices.

Toby's Tip: For a balanced breakfast, serve the Banana Walnut Protein Bread with plain nonfat Greek yogurt or a glass of ultra-filtered skim or reduced-fat milk on the side.

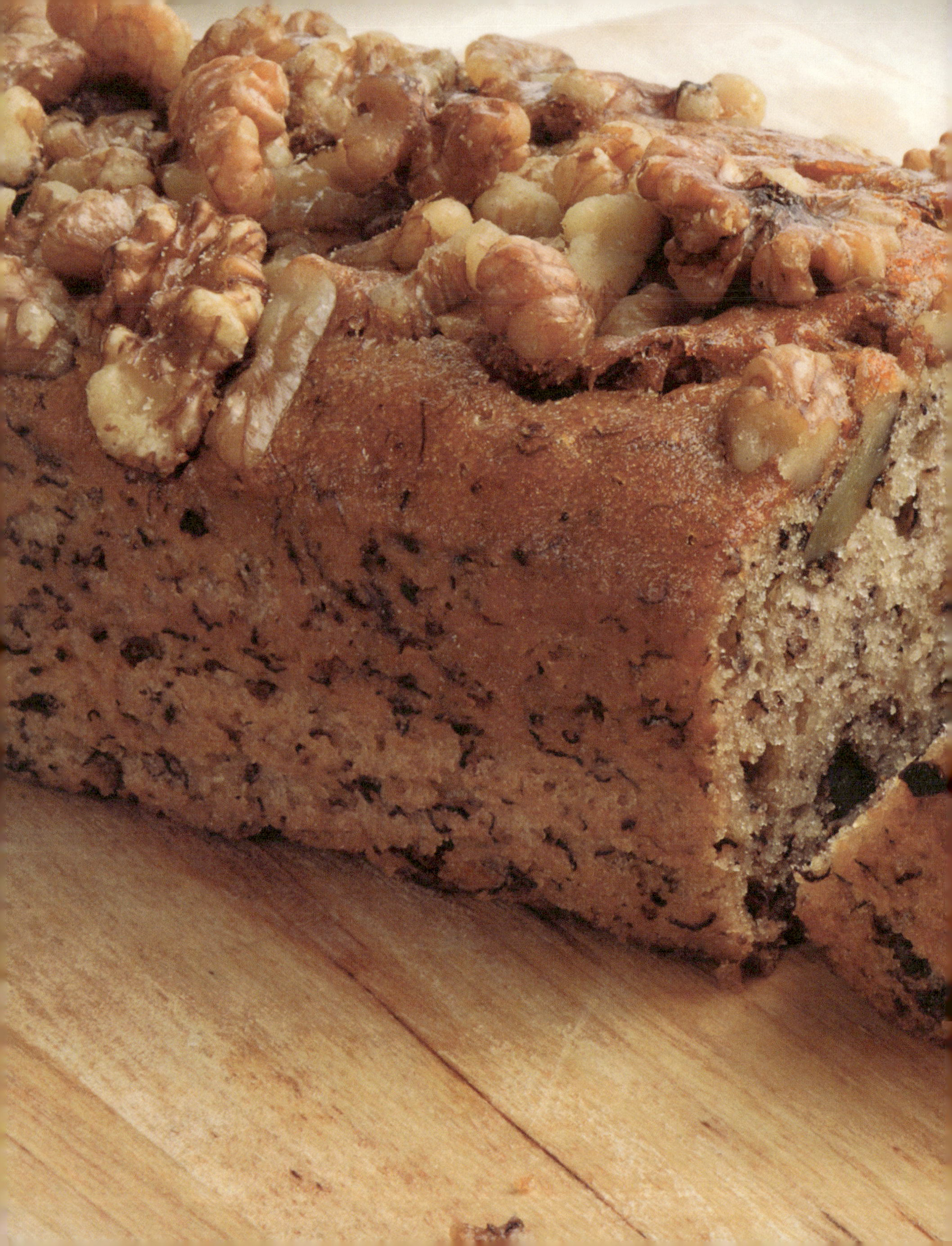

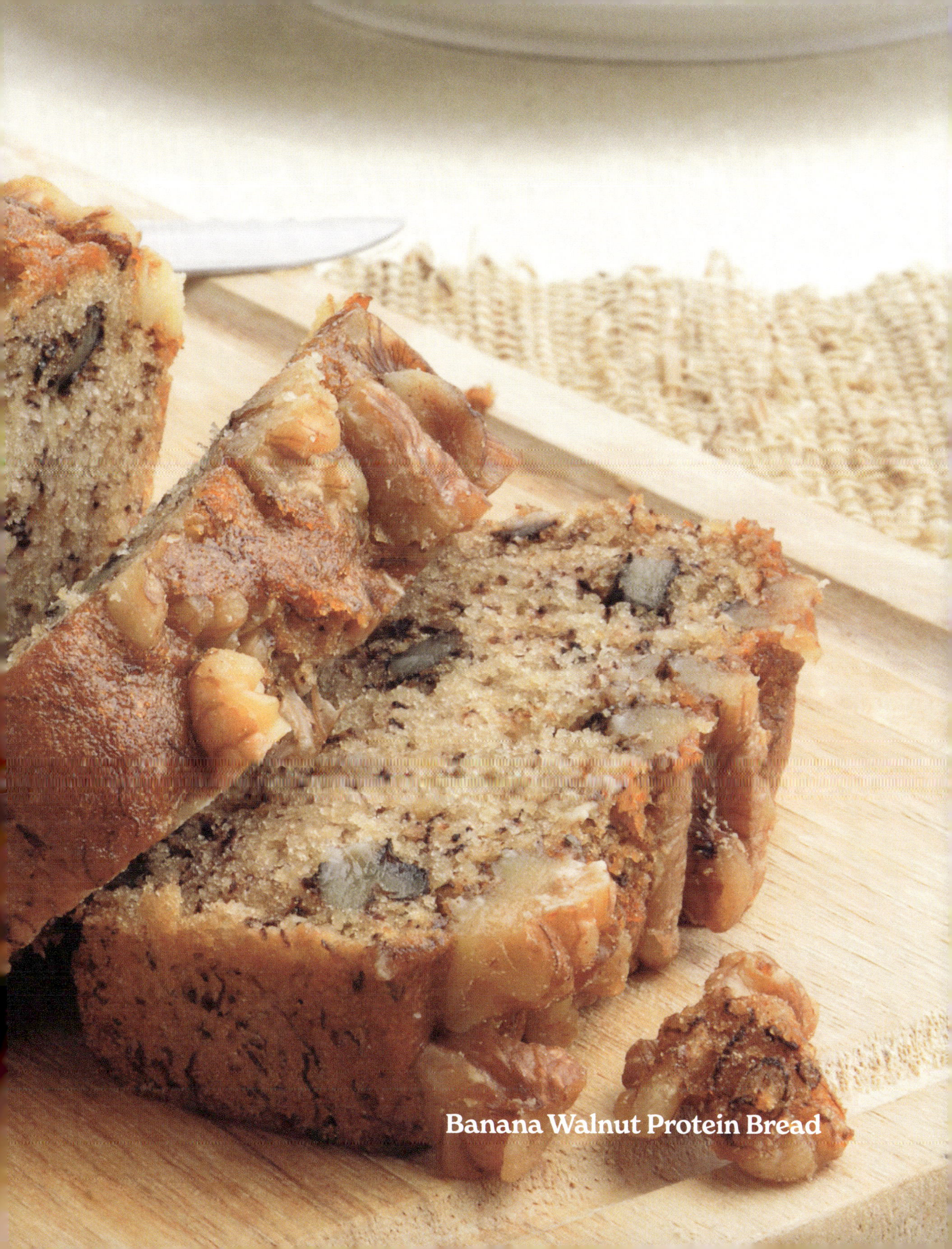

Banana Walnut Protein Bread

Pecan Pie Yogurt Bowl

For this yogurt bowl, you quickly whip up your own caramel, which is then drizzled over Greek yogurt and topped with pecans. The flavor is reminiscent of pecan pie but with more protein—a whopping 12 grams!

PREP TIME 10 min // **COOK TIME** 5 min // **TOTAL TIME** 15 min // **SERVINGS** 4 // **SERVING SIZE** 1 bowl

30 Minutes or Less | **Vegetarian, Gluten-Free**

- 5 tablespoons granulated sugar
- 2 tablespoons unsalted butter
- 3 tablespoons heavy whipping cream
- ½ teaspoon pure vanilla extract
- ⅛ teaspoon table salt
- 2 cups plain nonfat Greek yogurt, divided
- ¼ cup pecans, chopped, divided

1. Combine sugar and butter in a small saucepan. Place over low heat and cook, whisking continuously, until the mixture turns a light brown color, about 4 minutes. Add the heavy cream and whisk to combine. Once the steam has dissipated, stir rapidly for 1 full minute to combine the mixture. Then remove the pan from the heat and add in the vanilla and salt. Allow to cool for 5 minutes.
2. *To serve:* In each of four bowls, place ½ cup of the yogurt and stir about 2 tablespoons of caramel into each. Top with 1 tablespoon chopped pecans and serve.
3. *To meal prep*: In each of four containers, divide the yogurt and store the caramel and nuts separately. Cover and store in the refrigerator for up to 4 days.
4. *To reheat:* Microwave the caramel on high for 30 seconds and let stand for 2 minutes, then pour over yogurt before serving.

Nutrition Information (per serving): Calories 261; Total Fat 15g; Saturated Fat 8g; Protein 12g; Total Carbohydrates 20g; Fiber 1g; Total Sugars 19g (Includes Added Sugars 15g); Sodium 118mg

Toby's Tip: Swap the Greek yogurt for Skyr yogurt or cottage cheese.

Chocolate Protein Balls

Whether you want to call them protein balls, power balls, bliss balls, or energy bites, this bite-sized no-cook snack adds 9 grams of protein per 2-piece serving.

PREP TIME 20 min // **CHILL TIME** 20 min // **TOTAL TIME** 40 min // **SERVINGS** 6 // **SERVING SIZE** 2 bites

Meal Prep | **Vegetarian, Gluten-Free, Dairy-Free**

- 1 cup pitted Medjool dates
- ¾ cup rolled oats
- 6 tablespoons smooth peanut butter
- 2 tablespoons peanut butter powder (6 grams protein per serving)
- 2 tablespoons ground hemp seeds
- 2 tablespoons unsweetened cocoa
- ⅛ teaspoon kosher salt
- 2 tablespoons chopped unsalted dry-roasted peanuts
- 2 tablespoons semi-sweet chocolate chips

1. Place the dates in a blender. Cover and pulse a few times until the dates are roughly chopped. Add the oats, peanut butter, peanut butter powder, hemp seeds, cocoa, and salt; cover and pulse until the mixture is well combined and crumbly. Transfer the batter to a medium bowl.
2. To the bowl, add the peanuts and chocolate chips; mix to combine.
3. Using wet hands, roll a heaping tablespoon of batter into a 1½-inch ball; transfer to a clean plate. Repeat with the remaining batter (you should end up with 12 balls). Cover the plate and refrigerate for at least 20 minutes or up to 4 days.
4. *To meal prep:* Place 2 balls into each of six small resealable containers. Cover and refrigerate for up to 5 days.

Nutrition Information (per serving): Calories 290; Total Fat 14g; Saturated Fat 3g; Protein 9g; Total Carbohydrates 36g; Fiber 5g; Total Sugars 23g (Includes Added Sugars 3g); Sodium 116mg

Toby's Tip: Swap the peanuty ingredients (peanuts, peanut powder, and peanut butter) for their almond counterparts.

Cottage Cheese-Blueberry Muffins

It's not easy making a higher-protein muffin. If you add too much protein powder, the consistency becomes grainy. If you add pre-sweetened protein powder, the flavor can be off. Instead, you'll find that unsweetened whey protein isolate gives these muffins the perfect flavor and a whopping 12 grams of protein. Serve with 1 cup of ultra-filtered cow's milk or soy milk for an additional 13 grams and 8 grams, respectively.

PREP TIME 15 min // **COOK TIME** 20 min // **TOTAL TIME** 35 min // **SERVINGS** 12 // **SERVING SIZE** 1 muffin

Meal Prep | **Vegetarian**

Nonstick cooking spray

1 cup reduced-fat cottage cheese

1½ cups all-purpose flour

¼ cup rolled oats

2 (29-gram) scoops unflavored whey protein isolate (25 grams protein per 1 scoop)

2 teaspoons baking powder

1 teaspoon baking soda

¼ teaspoon table salt

¼ cup unsalted butter, softened

1½ tablespoons canola or safflower oil

¾ cup granulated sugar

2 large eggs, beaten

1 cup blueberries, fresh or frozen and thawed

1. Preheat the oven to 350°F. Coat a 12-cup muffin pan with nonstick cooking spray.
2. Place the cottage cheese in a blender and blend until smooth, about 1 minute. Set aside.
3. In a medium bowl, sift together the flour, oats, whey protein, baking powder, baking soda, and salt.
4. In a separate medium bowl, whisk together the cottage cheese, butter, and oil. Add the sugar and eggs, and whisk until the mixture is smooth.
5. Slowly add the dry ingredients to the wet ingredients, and mix using a wooden spoon, being careful not to overmix. Fold in the blueberries until incorporated.
6. Fill each muffin cup three-quarters with batter. Tap the muffin pan a few times on the counter to get rid of any bubbles.
7. Bake in the preheated oven until a toothpick placed into the center of 1 or 2 muffins comes out clean, about 20 minutes. Remove the muffin pan from the oven and allow the muffins to cool for 10 minutes. Then transfer the muffins to a wire rack and let cool completely.
8. *To meal prep:* Cover the muffins and store at room temperature for up to 5 days.

9. *To reheat*: Place a muffin on a microwave-safe plate and microwave on high for 30 seconds; let stand for 2 minutes to allow the heat to distribute evenly.

Nutrition Information (per serving): Calories 222; Total Fat 7g; Saturated Fat 3g; Protein 12g; Total Carbohydrates 29g; Fiber 1g; Total Sugars 14g (Includes Added Sugars 12.5g); Sodium 364mg

Toby's Tip: Swap the blueberries for 1 cup of sliced strawberries or raspberries, or 1 chopped apple or pear.

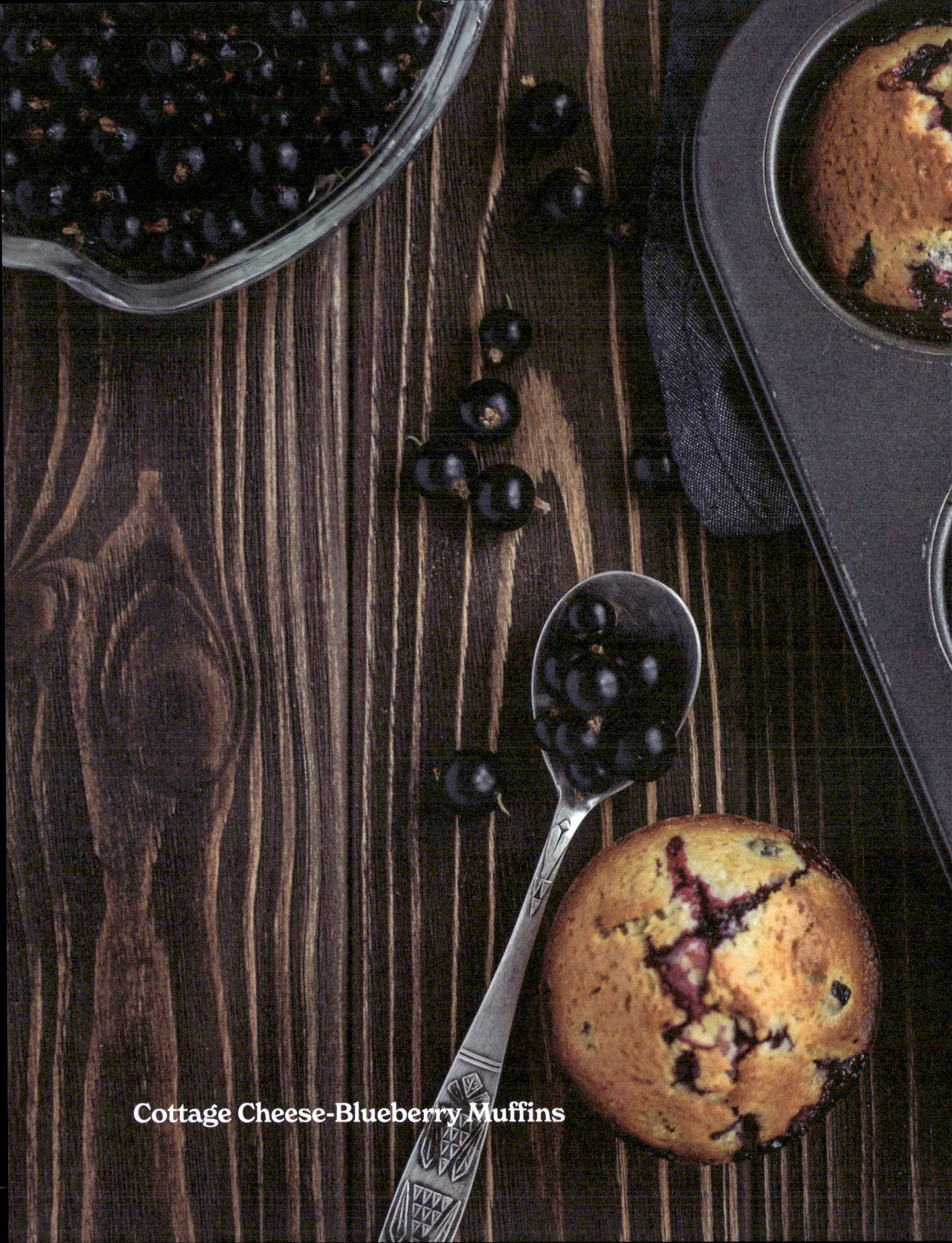

Cottage Cheese-Blueberry Muffins

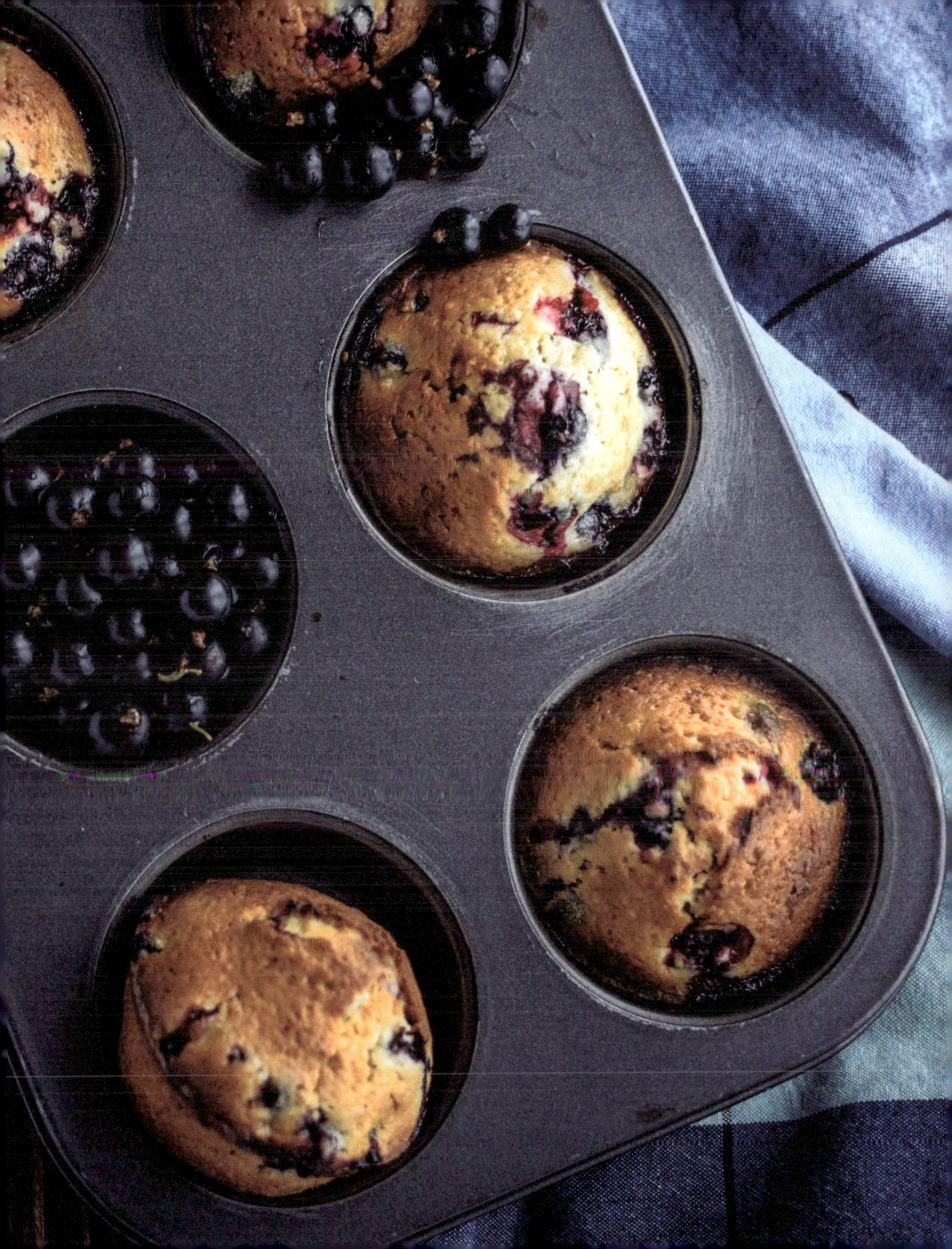

Panna Cotta *with* Strawberry-Chia Sauce

Instead of using heavy cream, this panna cotta uses Greek yogurt to maintain its creamy mouthfeel. When topped with the strawberry chia sauce, it provides a substantial 16 grams of protein per serving.

PREP TIME 4 hours, 50 min // **COOK TIME** 20 min // **TOTAL TIME** 5 hours, 10 min // **SERVINGS** 4
SERVING SIZE 1 dish

Meal Prep | **Vegetarian, Gluten-Free**

FOR THE PANNA COTTA

2 cups plain reduced-fat (2 percent) Greek yogurt

2 tablespoons granulated sugar

1 teaspoon pure vanilla extract

¾ cup ultra-filtered reduced-fat (2 percent) milk (13 grams protein per 1 cup serving)

2 teaspoons gelatin powder

FOR THE STRAWBERRY-CHIA SAUCE

2 cups sliced strawberries, fresh or frozen and defrosted

2 tablespoons chia seeds

1 tablespoon lemon juice

2 teaspoons liquid honey

1. *For the panna cotta:* In a medium bowl, mix together the yogurt, sugar, and vanilla. Set aside for 15 minutes to allow the mixture to come to room temperature.
2. Pour the milk into a cold, small saucepan and sprinkle the gelatin over top. Set aside for 5 minutes to let the gelatin soften.
3. Place the saucepan over low heat to warm the milk and melt the gelatin, being careful not to let it boil. Stir until the gelatin has melted, 1 to 2 minutes. Stir the warm milk into the yogurt mixture and combine thoroughly.
4. *To meal prep:* Pour about ½ cup of the mixture into each of four ramekins or small bowls. Cover with plastic wrap and refrigerate until set, at least 4 hours or up to 24 hours.
5. *For the strawberry chia sauce:* In a medium saucepan, add the strawberries and cook over medium heat until the strawberries begin to break down, about 10 minutes. Add the chia seeds, lemon juice, and liquid honey and toss to combine. Bring the mixture to a boil over high heat and then reduce the heat to medium-low and simmer, stirring occasionally, for 5 minutes. Remove the saucepan from the heat and allow to cool for 10 minutes.

6. *To serve:* Just before serving, spoon 2 tablespoons of the sauce over the panna cotta and enjoy. Sauce can be cool or served warm, right after cooking. Store in the refrigerator, covered, for up to 4 days.

Nutrition Information (per serving): Calories 213; Total Fat 5g; Saturated Fat 2g; Protein 16g; Total Carbohydrates 26g; Fiber 4g; Total Sugars 18g (Includes Added Sugars 9g); Sodium 136mg

Toby's Tip: Swap the peach compote from the Peach Compote Parfaits on page 126 for the Strawberry-Chia Sauce.

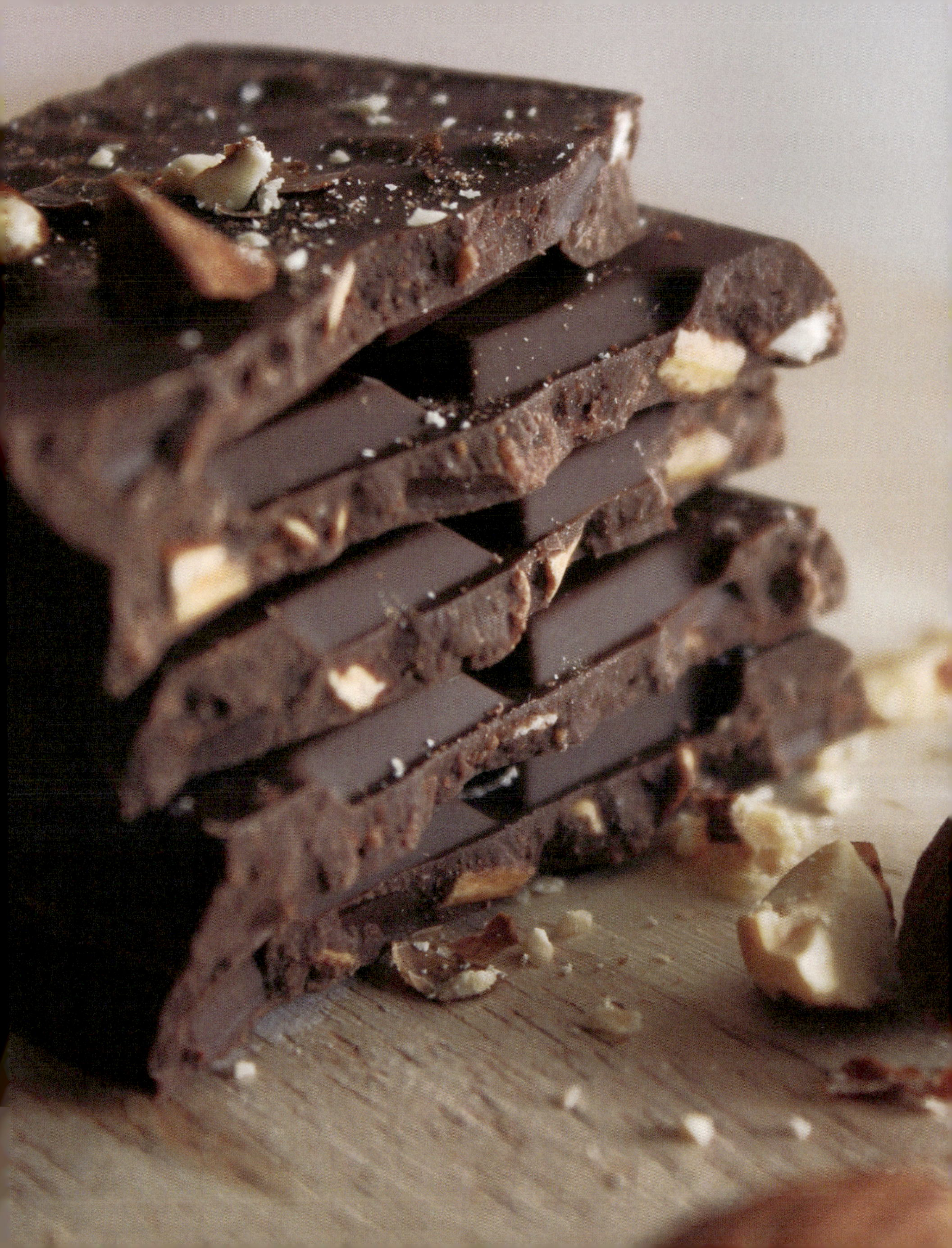

Chocolate Cottage Cheese Bark *with* Nuts

If you're a chocolate lover like me, you're always looking for a healthful way to satiate your chocolate craving. Look no further than this bark made with a combo of chocolate and cottage cheese and topped with nuts—it delivers 6 grams of protein per serving.

PREP TIME 2 hours, 20 min // **COOK TIME** 2 min // **TOTAL TIME** 2 hours, 22 min // **SERVINGS** 8

SERVING SIZE 2 pieces

Meal Prep, 30 Minutes or Less | **Vegetarian, Gluten-Free**

¾ cup reduced-fat (2 percent) cottage cheese

8 ounces 60 percent dark chocolate, broken into pieces

¼ cup unsalted dry-roasted almonds, chopped

¼ cup unsalted dry-roasted pistachios

⅛ teaspoon sea salt

Nutrition Information (per serving): Calories 230; Total Fat 15g; Saturated Fat 7g; Protein 6g; Total Carbohydrates 18g; Fiber 3g; Total Sugars 12g (Includes Added Sugars 10g); Sodium 96mg

1. Line a medium baking sheet with parchment paper. Set aside.
2. Place the cottage cheese in a blender. Cover and blend until smooth, about 1 minute. Let stand at room temperature for 15 minutes.
3. Place the chocolate pieces in a microwave-safe bowl and microwave on high for 30-second intervals, stirring thoroughly after each interval, until the chocolate has melted and is smooth, about 1½ minutes total. Set aside for 5 minutes to slightly cool.
4. Add the cottage cheese to the chocolate and stir until incorporated and smooth.
5. Spoon the chocolate mixture onto the prepared baking sheet. Using a spatula, spread the mixture evenly to the edges. Sprinkle evenly with the almonds, pistachios, and sea salt.
6. Transfer the baking sheet to the freezer for at least 2 hours, until the chocolate sets.
7. *To serve:* Break the bark into 16 pieces and serve. Store in a covered container in the refrigerator for up to 1 week.

Toby's Tip: Get creative and add more protein by sprinkling chia, hemp, pumpkin, or flax seeds too.

Layered Chocolate-Raspberry Popsicles

Popsicles aren't known for their high-protein content, but when you want a cooling sweet treat, *these* popsicles will do the trick. They're made with a layer of tart raspberries balanced with a protein- and chocolate-filled milk and ricotta layer, which provides a respectable 6 grams of protein per pop.

PREP TIME 4 hours, 17 min // **COOK TIME** 0 min // **TOTAL TIME** 4 hours, 17 min // **SERVINGS** 12

SERVING SIZE 1 popsicle

Meal Prep, Freezer-Friendly | **Vegetarian, Gluten-Free**

2 cups frozen raspberries

½ cup 100 percent pomegranate or cranberry juice

1 cup reduced-fat (2 percent) ultra-filtered chocolate milk (13 grams protein per 1 cup serving)

¼ cup whole-milk ricotta cheese

2 (25-gram) scoops whey protein isolate

2 tablespoons unsweetened cocoa

1 teaspoon pure vanilla extract

Nutrition Information (per serving): Calories 56; Total Fat 1g; Saturated Fat 1g; Protein 6g; Total Carbohydrates 6g; Fiber 1g; Total Sugars 3g (Includes Added Sugars 0.5g); Sodium 55mg

1. In a blender or food processor, add raspberries and juice. Cover and purée until smooth, about 1 minute. Transfer the mixture to a medium bowl and set aside. Rinse the blender or food processor and set aside for step 3.
2. Spoon about 2 tablespoons of the raspberry purée into each popsicle mold. Tap each mold on the counter several times to level the purée. Place in freezer for 15 minutes, until almost solid.
3. In the reserved blender, add the chocolate milk, ricotta cheese, protein powder, cocoa, and vanilla. Cover and blend on high speed until smooth, about 1 minute.
4. Remove the mold from freezer and spoon about 2 tablespoons of the chocolate mixture into molds. Return mold to the freezer. Freeze for at least 4 hours or until fully set.
5. *To serve:* Gently run cool water over the popsicle mold for 5 seconds to easily remove the popsicle from the mold.
6. *To meal prep*: Keep popsicles in their mold for up to 2 months.

Toby's Tip: If you choose to use fresh raspberries, blend and then strain through a cheesecloth to remove the seeds (unless you want them in your popsicle!).

APPENDIX

Protein per serving of common foods

Food	Portion	Protein (grams)
MEAT, POULTRY, FISH		
Beef, chicken, turkey, pork, lamb	1 ounce	7
Beef or turkey jerky	1 ounce	10 to 15
Seafood (crabmeat, shrimp, lobster)	1 ounce	6
MEAT, POULTRY, FISH		
Soy milk	8 fluid ounces	7
Edamame (shelled and cooked)	½ cup	8
Tofu	1 ounce	3
SEEDS		
Hemp hearts	1 tablespoon	3
Chia seeds	1 tablespoon	3
Flax seeds	1 tablespoon	2
Pumpkin seeds	1 tablespoon	1
Sunflower seeds	1 ounce	5
NUTS		
Peanuts (dry roasted)	2 tablespoons	4
Almonds (dry roasted)	2 tablespoons	4
Walnuts (halves)	2 tablespoons	2
Pine nuts	2 tablespoons	2
Pistachios (dry roasted)	2 tablespoons	3
Peanut butter, smooth or chunky	2 tablespoons	7
Almond milk	8 fluid ounces	1
MILK AND DAIRY FOODS		
Feta (crumbled)	2 tablespoons	3
Goat cheese (crumbled)	1 ounce	4 to 6 (depending on brand)

Food	Portion	Protein (grams)
Part-skim mozzarella (shredded)	2 tablespoons	4
Parmesan (grated)	2 tablespoons	4
Reduced-fat cheddar (shredded)	2 tablespoons	4
Cottage cheese	½ cup	About 14
Icelandic yogurt (skyr)	5.3 ounces	14 to 18
Milk, fat-free or 1 percent low fat	8 fluid ounces	8
Milk, ultra-filtered	8 fluid ounces	13
Greek yogurt	5 ounces	12 to 18
Kefir	1 cup	10
VEGAN CHEESE ALTERNATIVE		
Nutritional yeast	2 tablespoons	5
BEANS, PEAS, LENTILS		
Chickpeas (canned)	½ cup	5
Black beans (canned)	½ cup	6
Lentils, brown (cooked)	½ cup	9
Cannellini beans (canned)	½ cup	8
Kidney beans (canned)	½ cup	8
Green peas (frozen)	½ cup	4
Hummus	¼ cup	7
QUICK PROTEINS		
Rotisserie chicken (skinless)	3 ounces	24
Hard-boiled egg	1 large	6
Canned sardines (packed in water)	4.4-ounce can (can sizes vary)	25
Canned chicken breast (packed in water)	3 ounces (drained)	15
Canned chunk light tuna (packed in water)	3 ounces (drained)	20
Canned salmon (packed in water)	3 ounces (drained)	18

INDEX

ACKNOWLEDGMENTS

I want to thank the team of people who made this book possible. Always first is my talented literary agent, Sally Ekus, who has stood by my side for more than ten years. Also, a big thank-you to my editor, Jenny Croghan, who always promotes positivity to create the best work possible. I would also like to thank my assistant and fellow registered dietitian, Amanda Godman, who is always most helpful to work with.

A big thank-you to the book designer and art director, John Calmeyer, and publicity and marketing expert Chris Fann.

Last, I would like to thank my three children, who I love very much. Now that I am an empty nester, I don't have my daughters to help me test and taste recipes or my son to eat the extra food. However, I do want to thank them for being independent young adults who are growing up and allowing me the time to write this cookbook.

ABOUT THE AUTHOR

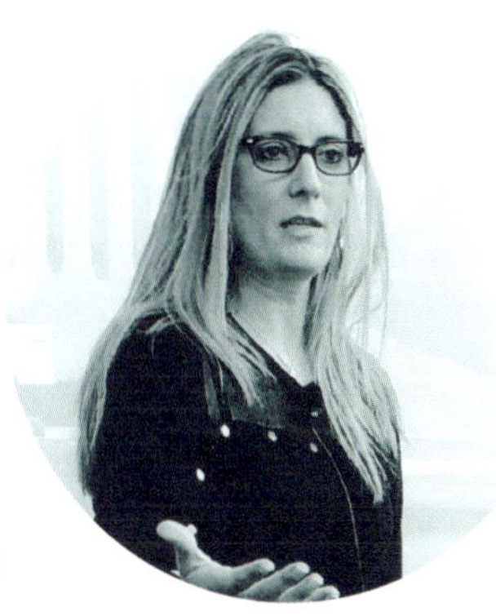

Toby Amidor, MS, RD, CDN, FAND is the founder of Toby Amidor Nutrition, PC, where she provides nutrition and food safety consulting services for individuals, restaurants, and food brands. She is a *Wall Street Journal*–bestselling cookbook author and has eleven published cookbooks. For close to 20 years Toby has been the nutrition expert for FoodNetwork.com, and founding contributor to their Healthy Eats blog. Toby is a regular contributor to many national online publications and for more than a decade has been penning the "Ask the Expert" column in *Today's Dietitian* magazine. She is also on the medical board for Forbes.com and EatThis.com and on the editorial board for *Today's Dietitian* magazine. As a nutrition expert, she has been quoted in hundreds of publications and regularly appears on local and national television shows. Toby is an adjunct professor at Quinnipiac University. For 11 years Toby was an adjunct professor at Teachers College, Columbia University teaching food service management and also taught at CUNY Hunter School of Public Urban Health and Lehman College in NYC.

Toby trained as a clinical dietitian at New York University. Through ongoing consulting and faculty positions, she has established herself as one of the top experts in culinary nutrition, food safety, and media communications. In 2018, Toby was awarded by the Academy of Nutrition & Dietetics the coveted Media Excellence Award.

ENDNOTES

1. International Food Information Council, "2025 Food and Health Survey" (Washington, DC: IFIC Foundation, October 2025), https://ific.org/wp-content/uploads/IFIC-FH-Survey-Food-Nutrition-October-2025.pdf.
2. U.S. Department of Agriculture and U.S. Department of Health and Human Services, Dietary Guidelines for Americans, 2020–2025, 9th ed. (Washington, DC: U.S. Government Publishing Office, December 2020), https://www.dietaryguidelines.gov/sites/default/files/2020-12/Dietary_Guidelines_for_Americans_2020-2025.pdf.

ABOUT CIDER MILL PRESS

Cider Mill Press publishes exceptional books that combine creativity and craftsmanship. As an imprint of HarperCollins Focus, we specialize in premium cookbooks, cocktail and spirits guides, and illustrated gift books, all distinguished by compelling content, striking design, and a commitment to quality in every detail. Cider Mill Press sets the standard for books that inform, inspire, and elevate everyday moments. Learn more at cidermillpress.com.

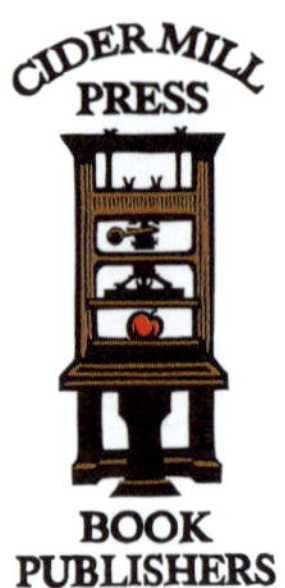

"Where Good Books Are Ready for Press"
501 Nelson Place
Nashville, Tennessee 37214 USA